Schizophre
Fate of the _ _...

International Perspectives in Philosophy and Psychiatry

Series editors: Bill (K.W.M.) Fulford, Katherine Morris, John Z Sadler, and Giovanni Stanghellini

Volumes in the series:

Forthcoming volumes in the series:

Schizophrenia and the Fate of the Self

Paul H. Lysaker

and

John T. Lysaker

OXFORD
UNIVERSITY PRESS

OXFORD
UNIVERSITY PRESS

Great Clarendon Street, Oxford OX2 6DP

Oxford University Press is a department of the University of Oxford.
It furthers the University's objective of excellence in research, scholarship,
and education by publishing worldwide in

Oxford New York

Auckland Cape Town Dar es Salaam Hong Kong Karachi
Kuala Lumpur Madrid Melbourne Mexico City Nairobi
New Delhi Shanghai Taipei Toronto

With offices in

Argentina Austria Brazil Chile Czech Republic France Greece
Guatemala Hungary Italy Japan Poland Portugal Singapore
South Korea Switzerland Thailand Turkey Ukraine Vietnam

Oxford is a registered trade mark of Oxford University Press
in the UK and in certain other countries

Published in the United States
by Oxford University Press Inc., New York

© Oxford University Press 2008

A catalogue record for this title is available from the British Library
Data available

Library of Congress Cataloguing in Publication Data
Data available

Typeset by Cepha Imaging Private Ltd., Bangalore, India
Printed in Great Britain
on acid-free paper by
Biddles Ltd., King's Lynn, UK

ISBN 978–0–19–921576–8

10 9 8 7 6 5 4 3 2 1

For Yvonne Lysaker, and in memory of
Richard Lysaker, from two most fortunate sons.

Preface

Recent systematic research has tended to regard schizophrenia as an expression of aberrant biology and the impact of social injustice on the vulnerable. With advances in medical technology and with many large-scale, longitudinal studies now underway, social and biological science have built a convincing case that the varieties of madness subsumed by the label schizophrenia are created, fueled and sustained by genetic, biochemical and environmental factors.

While this literature represents an advance, it can have the effect of leading us to lose track of those who experience, interpret and live with schizophrenia. With ever more detailed models of the neurobiological and social systems out of which schizophrenia is born, it is possible to overlook how suffering persons experience their symptoms. One might also miss how they value or frame the challenges their conditions pose and navigate their way through life, that is seek security, companionship, and meaning. Our goal is to attend to and help articulate the root experiences of persons who suffer from schizophrenia. More particularly, we hope to discuss some of the disorder's key, first-person dimensions, and in a way that not only avoids dualism, but both illuminates some of schizophrenia's clinical and psychosocial dimensions, and provides concrete directions for treatment.

The first two chapters will provide a series of general reviews regarding schizophrenia. The basic features of schizophrenia will be outlined and prevailing theories about the biological and social forces that significantly contribute to the onset and course of the illness will be summarized. Next, observations from multiple perspectives about the subjective experience of schizophrenia will be detailed. When read together, these observations suggest that persons with schizophrenia often experience themselves diminishing over the course of their illness, as if their presence and effectiveness in their lives were less than it had been.

Given their generality and focus on review, these first two sections may contain discussion already familiar to certain readers. However, they should be of interest to those less familiar with the vast literature on schizophrenia. Moreover, both chapters contain discussions that are integral to our argument that the first-person dimensions of schizophrenia merit closer and more sustained attention. Even those familiar with the literature surrounding schizophrenia may find them of interest, therefore.

In Chapter 3, we offer a theory of the self in preparation for an account of how someone might come to experience him or herself as diminished in schizophrenia. Our view is essentially dialogical. We suggest that human beings exist as ongoing interpersonal and intrapersonal exchanges or dialogues that emerge as responses to shifting worldly contexts, and which reflect complementary as well as dissonant facets of our being. Now, to say that we *are* these responsive dialogues, is to claim that human being entails webs of physiological dispositions, acquired roles, and evolving self-presentations, which cannot be properly understood as the modes of an enduring substance or the acts of a univocal agency.

On the basis of these first three chapters, we then turn to our principal concern: an account of some key first-person aspects of schizophrenia, which the next four chapters explore via the following questions. First, do disruptions in those dialogical processes that appear to enable sense of self help us account for the kinds of self-experiences that, over the last hundred years, have been associated with schizophrenia? Furthermore, does our dialogical account tell us anything new about how to understand these disturbances? Next, we consider whether a dialogical account of schizophrenia's first-person dimensions might help us understand the emergence of a range of symptoms. And can it do so without presuming another version of mind–body dualism? Third, we explore whether a dialogical account of first-person experience might also help us understand the persistence of psychosocial dysfunction in schizophrenia. Does systematic reflection on self-experience help us understand challenges, widely found among persons with schizophrenia, which make it difficult to richly and effectively engage oneself and the world? Finally, we turn to the question of whether a dialogical account of first-person experience has any implications for the treatment of others. Does a dialogical conception of schizophrenia's first-person dimensions, particularly when integrated with some of the disorder's objective features, help individual psychotherapy enable persons to live more effectively with their illness and its attendant difficulties?

Like any book of this length, our study has benefited from the support and insights of several others. Giancarlo Dimaggio and Hubert Hermans provided support and guidance with regard to the shape of the book and our more general involvement with dialogical theories of the self. They are exceptionally fine colleagues, and we are grateful for their friendship. Valerie LaRocco, with care and skill, helped extensively by proof-reading chapters and compiling references. Kelly Buck was an active partner in many discussions regarding the psychotherapy of schizophrenia. Aaron Mishira shared work and information that helped us frame our discussion of the phenomenological conception of self-disturbance. David Roe provided helpful insight and information regarding the rehabilitation point of view of self-disturbance. Mark Johnson read and offered useful suggestions regarding Chapter 3, and both he and Scott Pratt were ongoing interlocutors with regard to these matters. Sara Hodges, Bertram Malle, Don Tucker and a group of graduate students from the University of Oregon Psychology Department, read and discussed these issues, in ways that proved helpful. As the bibliography will show, several journals published papers that presented our views at various stages of development. Thanks to them and the readers who reviewed our submissions. Also, many audiences have heard bits and pieces along the way. Their enthusiastic reception of our many starts and revisions has been a real incentive to systematize our view in a single, prolonged study. Paul Lysaker would also like to thank the Abbey Coffee House in Indianapolis, Indiana where he did much of his writing. John Lysaker would like to thank T. K. McDonald, whose reliable presence and good humor allowed him to devote most of his summer energy to working on the manuscript.

Of course, more than professional colleagues and friends sustain intellectual work. Paul Lysaker would like to thank his beloved wife

Judy, who provided not only patience and support but also wisdom and insight which directly inspired and informed much of the thinking of this book. Many of the thoughts in this book are most inextricably entwined with her ideas and thus are a reflection of her own deep thinking. Paul Lysaker would also like to thank his beloved daughter Mercedes Lysaker for her unwavering love and for her young but rigorous and questioning mind which was a source of inspiration. John Lysaker would like to thank his dear, dear Hilary Hart for many, many things. Her companionship is a source of energy, and her loving and enthusiastic support for this and similar ventures makes pursuing them more rewarding than they otherwise would be. He is particularly grateful for her patience during the year of 2007, when this project left him occasionally distracted and self-absorbed, or in other words, not very much fun.

Finally, no one moves very far in life without gifts bestowed by parents. The authors are more grateful than words for the life, love, and ongoing support of Yvonne and Richard Lysaker. Thanks also to our other siblings, Eric and Jill for their good humor and support throughout the years. Irreverent sons can be a burden, but our parents bore it with a wit and grace more than equal to the task. Moreover, they never wavered in their enthusiasm for our intellectual pursuits, and few children in this commercial age have enjoyed that blessing. We thus dedicate this book to our mother, Yvonne Lysaker, and to the memory of our father, Richard Lysaker, and we do so with the sure sense that without them, our lives, let alone this exhilarating collaboration, would not have been possible.

Contents

Chapter 1

Symptoms and common explanations

As much as any medical illness, schizophrenia presents sufferers, their families, communities, scientists, thinkers and practitioners with an enormous array of social, biological and economic conundrums. It also confronts us with profound human suffering, for it involves alterations in the core of a person's subjectivity. The phenomenon of schizophrenia, which can be found in widely divergent cultures and multiple historical eras, thus compels our attention for several reasons. First and foremost, it is saturated with human pain and need, and one cannot help but to wonder how best to address the anguish that is its hallmark. Schizophrenia also seems to open a path into how the brain facilitates conscious awareness, how social networks form and function, and how interpersonal relations form and sustain a sense of self. And it raises stark questions regarding social responsibility for the disenfranchised, particularly given how poorly the West has sometimes treated the mentally ill. Then it makes one wonder about what should lie at the heart of psychological treatments that aim to meliorate human suffering. Schizophrenia thus opens us to ourselves at the individual and social level, and in ways that concern natural scientists, social scientists, and humanists alike. As Jenkins (2004) noted: 'schizophrenia itself offers a paradigm case for scientific understandings of culturally fundamental and ordinal processes and capacities of the self, the emotions and social engagement' (p. 29). Barham (1993) observed that it requires us to define and redefine the meanings of the common and the 'bounds of community' (p. 198).

Before presenting and pursuing the key task for this volume, which is an exploration of self-experience in schizophrenia, we wish to establish a context for our explorations. In particular, we will clarify what we mean by schizophrenia and summarize much of what is generally associated with it. This chapter will present the canonical definitions of schizophrenia, as well as summary explanations of when it begins, what may cause it, and how it develops and unfolds over the course of a life.

As widely noted by proponents and critics of schizophrenia research, the number of pages in newly published papers and book chapters on schizophrenia is enormous. A casual guess is that it approaches or exceeds 500 pages of possibly relevant material per month. A comprehensive review of research of the last decade would consequently require several volumes. Our overview will take many shortcuts, therefore, and risk certain generalities. Foremost among the latter will be our presentation of schizophrenia as a singular concept. In truth, schizophrenia probably refers to several conditions that share common features and present a relatively common set of dilemmas, but which develop along divergent paths. As noted by Bleuler (1911/1950), who coined the term a hundred years ago, it is a group of conditions that may have different antecedents.

Our initial survey views schizophrenia in terms of the violent collision of biological forces and/or social forces within the space of an individual life. It is thus decidedly not polemical. Instead, we wish to orient our reader to how schizophrenia is commonly defined, attending to its characteristic symptoms, onset, and possible courses. We then organize and present a range of empirical research in order to articulate the common dilemmas faced by those who suffer from schizophrenia, beginning with neurobiological accounts of what is sometimes popularly called 'the broken brain'. We then look at suggestions that unjust and destructive social and cultural processes are in part responsible for the onset and disabilities of schizophrenia. After this review, we will begin to argue that schizophrenia also retains an irreducible, first-person dimension, and that an adequate conception of the disorder must track the fate of sense of self over the course of the illness.

Schizophrenia: general characteristics

Symptoms

Schizophrenia is not a rare condition. One out of every hundred people experiences it, and that holds for industrial and Third World countries.

It occurs in various ways and to various degrees, and so 'schizophrenia' is ultimately a descriptor signifying a collection of experiences. It is a diagnosis based on observations that indicate the presence or absence of a number of specific perceptions, behaviors, thoughts or emotions that evolve over a period of many months.

As defined in the United States by the *Diagnostic and Statistical Manual (DSM) IV-TR* of the American Psychiatric Association (2000), to qualify for a diagnosis of schizophrenia a person must exhibit at least two from a list of five characteristic symptoms. The first of these characteristic symptoms are delusions. Delusions involve odd, even bizarre thoughts that most everyone finds incredulous. Examples of delusions commonly encountered include thinking that one's relatives are poisoning one, that one is an heir to a multi-billion dollar fortune, that one is close friends with a national leader, that shifting traffic patterns hold special messages, that one's heart is a stone, and that earlier in life one was raised on an island by radioactive sharks. Or consider this. A man walks into a lobby and sees a woman laughing. He finds her laughter overwhelming and unpleasant to listen to and becomes convinced that this laughter is a signal for the police to arrest and imprison him.

The second set of characteristic symptoms are hallucinations, sensory perceptions not shared by others. Together with delusions, they form a set of 'positive symptoms' because they represent the presence of experiences not shared by most. Hallucinations can involve voices or sounds, vivid visual images, pungent odors, and/or bodily sensations, each of which appears to lack a discernable external cause. People may hear voices from a loudspeaker viciously criticizing them publicly, see devils sitting atop a sink, hear popular music coming from their stomach, hear a voice telling them to buy fried chicken, and smell foul and decaying things while attending an Alcoholics Anonymous meeting.

A third characteristic symptom that would contribute to a diagnosis of schizophrenia involves disorganized speech, or speech without clear or even apparent connections among ideas. Within a single sentence a person might refer to his or her mother, the roughness versus the smoothness of cloth, and the bitterness of coffee, and without any apparent connection between any two of these thoughts. A man, within half a minute, speaking without interruption or apparent punctuation, might refer to a routine visit to a dentist, a chipped filling, a steel needle, x-rays, Africans in general, being poisoned, not being allowed emotions, saline solution, sex, crying, queasy feelings in his stomach, and Vietnam.

The fourth set of characteristic symptoms entail disorganized or catatonic behavior, which is to say, acting in ways that are frenetic and chaotic, without any apparent purpose, or having no behavior at all – just standing or sitting as if frozen. A person in a catatonic state might rigidly sit for an hour with a blank expression, as if made out of plastic.

Negative symptoms form a fifth set of characteristic symptoms, and involve the absence of essential capacities that help people remain linked with the world. Examples include the loss of interest in others. Not that one fears others and so avoids them: rather, one simply shows no interest in socializing. Or, there may be an apparent lack of emotion or desire. As a man cogently explained to us several years ago, his true disability lay in being completely unable to direct his life in any manner. Another explained that he lived in a 'cloudbank'. Each day, he had little sense of what he felt or wanted.

While schizophrenia thus signifies a range of unusual and frightening symptoms from across these five categories, a diagnosis of schizophrenia also requires significant degrees of social, community or occupational dysfunction, which must represent a decline from previous levels of function. A person who previously worked might now be unable to hold a job. A person who had close friends and used to date might now have few if any social contacts. Importantly, the duration of these disturbances must also be considered before a person can be described as experiencing or having schizophrenia. According to the DSM-IV-TR, there must be continuous signs of disturbance for at least 6 months, and the characteristic symptoms must have lasted for one month, unless treated. As might be expected, the symptoms must not result from intoxication or drug abuse/dependence. Nor should they be an effect of depressed or manic states, or be attributable to a distinct medical condition. People who hear or see things that others do not, or who have profoundly disorganized behavior due to a brain tumor, drug intoxication or severe grief, should not be diagnosed as suffering from schizophrenia.

Subtypes and comorbidities

Given its wide range of symptoms, it is unsurprising that many attempts have been made to determine specific subtypes or forms of schizophrenia. The most popular are those offered by the DSM-IV-TR. Although their validity is still being assessed, their conception dates back over 100 years to Bleuler's original classification of subgroups, and they are commonly used in clinical settings. 'Paranoid schizophrenia', often invoked in the media as the most desperate form of madness, is one of the DSM subtypes. Ironically, it actually describes people whose cognition is generally intact but who suffer prominent hallucinations and delusions. The *disorganized* type, by contrast, describes people whose primary difficulties involve cognitive disorganization, whereas the *undifferentiated* type, another DSM subtype, describes people who suffer from both hallucinations and/or delusions and disorganization.

Another approach to understanding whether there are categories of schizophrenia has distinguished between 'deficit' and 'non-deficit' schizophrenia (e.g. Kirkpatrick and Buchanan, 1990). According to this hypothesis, there is a discrete group of people with schizophrenia who have the 'deficit syndrome', that is, who experience negative symptoms such as lack of interest, emotion, or volition over a period of years, and this is the primary manifestation of their condition. Predictably, the negative symptoms must not result from other factors such as medication side-effects, hallucinations, delusions or depression. Moreover, positive symptoms should not characterize the condition. Thus, people who persistently withdraw from others and display a very limited range of affect due to a belief that others want to kill them should not be described as experiencing the deficit syndrome. However, someone who has been unable to experience pleasure for years, and who has had no desire to interact with others could be described as suffering from the deficit syndrome.

Beyond the key symptoms of schizophrenia, it should also be noted that there are a variety of other problems that frequently occur among people with schizophrenia. Some of these may be related to biological aspects of the condition and others to lifestyles sometimes correlated with it. For instance, the risk of serious medical illnesses including heart disease, diabetes and obesity is elevated in schizophrenia (Goff *et al.*, 2005). As many as a third to a half of people with schizophrenia may also be strikingly unaware of or deny what others perceive as their deficits and difficulties (Amador *et al.*, 1994). They may doggedly persist in the belief there is nothing wrong in their lives and/or that they need no help. There is also a significantly increased rate of legal problems (Lamb and Weinberger, 1998), homelessness (Bachrach, 1992), as well as substance abuse and dependence in the population (Mueser *et al.*, 1990). Schizophrenia is also linked to a relatively high incidence of anxiety, dysphoria, and maladaptive patterns of relating to others (Pallanti, Quercioli and Hollander, 2004; Solano and Chavez, 2000). Similarly, emotional misery is more the rule that the exception. The vast majority of people with schizophrenia (approximately 75 percent) also struggle to work steadily, even when provided with aggressive vocational rehabilitation programs (Bond, Drake, Mueser and Becker, 1997). In general, then, suffering and disadvantage of all kinds seems to accompany this condition.

Onset and prevalence

As symptoms vary between people, so can the manner and timing with which they emerge. For some, the disorder occurs abruptly. For instance, within a period of two months, a man in his early twenties who we will call Frank, went from a life of work and extensive social connections to being homebound and riddled with the fear of being assassinated. One month he was working and having coffee with friends. Two months later, he could speak of nothing other than the danger he faced every moment. In late adolescence, another man slipped from being an exceptional math student to a student struggling to pass every class. He slowly withdrew from friends, developed a cannabis addiction, and finally withdrew from school. He later tried to function as a soldier in the military, a material handler, and then a roadie for a rock band. Eventually he concluded that he could not trust anyone and became homeless. Two years after his initial troubles, he found himself in a nursing home, 500 miles away from home, recovering from injuries sustained when he was beaten unconscious by police officers who thought he was drunk. In that nursing home he hallucinated a chorus of surrounding angels and devils, and continued to do so for decades.

Regarding who develops schizophrenia and how long its conditions last, several long-standing beliefs recently have been challenged. For instance, schizophrenia was once considered a disorder that develops between late adolescence and the mid-thirties, as in the cases just mentioned. It is now believed, however, that it is not uncommon for the illness to first appear in adults over the age of forty-five (Jeste, Symonds and Harris, 1997). It can also occur in children, although rarely (Asarnow, Thompson and McGrath, 2004). Men and women are also affected differently, and different kinds of links between onset and outcome affect each population. For example, women tend to have relatively later onset than men. However, earlier onset for men appears linked to poorer long-term outcomes, while women who experience earlier onset may alternately face better prognoses (Lewine, Haden, Caudel and Shurett, 1997).

Schizophrenia was also long thought of as an egalitarian disorder that affects people regardless of their gender, race or socioeconomic status. This also has been challenged. McGrath and colleagues (2004) gathered over 100 studies conducted between 1965 and 2001. All told, 33 countries are represented in this group. Looking at original data related to the incidence of schizophrenia, McGrath and colleagues concluded that contrary to long-standing beliefs, not everyone had the same relative risk of developing schizophrenia. For instance, males appeared to have a significantly higher rate of schizophrenia relative to females (2.4 vs. 0.9 percent). Immigrants also experienced dramatically greater rates of schizophrenia than natives (12.8 vs. 1.0 percent).

Course of illness

It has been thoroughly documented that symptom levels can fluctuate dramatically over time, moving from acute periods to others in which they appear to vanish. A man we know shows precisely this. Previously married and employed for years, he became ill. One day, he would attribute his actions to commands sent to him through electrical currents by non-corporeal spirits. A month later, he could coherently talk about his past and future, and argue that there was no reason to defend his previous beliefs about spirits. A month after this, he destroyed the furniture in his apartment and stopped eating to punish the spirits who he again believed directed his actions. Two months after brawling with his furniture, beliefs concerning spirits were gone and he reorganized his life. Four months following that, he was arrested for stealing items from a local department store. He claimed that he needed the items for a ritual that would honor the spirits who controlled his actions. As one can see, symptoms are stable traits, but they can fluctuate dramatically over short periods of time.

While it is recognized that symptom severity can change from time to time, it remains a matter of considerable debate whether, and if so, how often, people thoroughly and enduringly recapture their health. One point of view, well summarized in 1992 by Harding and colleagues, suggests that the majority of people with schizophrenia recover in some meaningful manner. These authors review a variety of long-term, longitudinal studies of outcome in both the United States and Europe, which interviewed people with histories of schizophrenia (or surviving family members) many years after inpatient treatment. A meticulously conducted study in Vermont was among those reviewed. It determined outcomes following exhaustive follow-up for 118 people diagnosed as severely ill and treated in a Vermont state hospital. Among these 118 people, the average period of time from hospitalization to follow-up was 32 years. The study suggested that roughly two-thirds of inpatients diagnosed with some form of schizophrenia demonstrated recovery or significant improvement. Harding compared this to European studies that followed even larger numbers of people for intervals of over 20 years. These studies also reported significant improvement rates in more than 50 percent of those diagnosed with schizophrenia.

In contrast, other studies report far lower rates of meaningful recovery (Harrow, Grossman, Herbener and Davies, 2000; Herbener, Harrow and Hill, 2005). These examinations of routine follow-ups 10–20 years after treatment show fluctuations in symptom levels but, in most cases, no significant improvements. In particular, these studies report that roughly only one-fifth of the sample appeared to attain a significant freedom from symptoms. What are we to make of this? Torgalsboen and Rund (1998) have studied far fewer people over smaller periods of time, but uniquely, they have included detailed accounts of individuals' perceptions of their condition. They found that many in their sample experienced fluctuating courses with distinct period of remission, followed by cyclical periods of lesser degrees of wellness. They suggest that schizophrenia is naturally neither a matter of slow deterioration or linear movement towards wellness but instead follows a fluctuating course, which is dictated by an individual's psychological make-up and the unpredictable twists of fate.

In our view, this range of disagreement suggests that schizophrenia follows out widely varying courses and meets with equally varying outcomes. On the one hand, it is widely cited that one in ten people suffering from schizophrenia commit suicide, and at least twice that many attempt suicide at least once during their illness (Torrey, 2001). That said, even among the most disordered people, some will meaningfully improve, and thus one would be mistaken to take a largely pessimistic viewpoint regarding outcome.

Schizophrenia: common explanations

Aberrant biology

Whatever schizophrenia is, most agree that it was first conceptualized nearly 100 years ago in the works of Bleuler (1911/1950) and Kraeplin (1919/2002). Together these authors are credited with documenting and linking the disturbances now regarded as characteristic symptoms of schizophrenia. They also suggested, implicitly and explicitly, that the phenomena apparent in so many asylums across Europe resulted from diseases of the brain and central nervous system. Bleuler argued that many of the dilemmas observed in his patients made sense as emergent inabilities of the brain to link ideas to one another. While he conceded that a person's issues or 'complexes' could be exaggerated by the disorder, that multiple outcomes were possible, and that the organic roots of the disturbance had yet to be determined, he regarded the illness as a 'cerebral disease'. He systematically denied that social or psychological factors were possible causes. Kraeplin, who referred to schizophrenia as Dementia Praecox, was even more direct in his insistence. On his view, he was observing the slowly diminishing capacities of the brain to either direct action or find pleasure or interest in the world. For Kraeplin, schizophrenia is a progressive brain disease that begins early in adulthood and has a steadily worsening course which ends in wholly encompassing dementia. From the beginning, therefore, schizophrenia has been cast as the breakdown of fundamental, biological processes whose corruption undermines the agency and coherence of individual lives.

Over the last several decades, no perspective has held greater sway over schizophrenia research than biological psychiatry. Returning to some of the basic observations or attitudes of Bleuler and Kraeplin and fueled by technological advances as well as millions upon millions of dollars in research funds, an international field of researchers, for several years, has been systematically examining schizophrenia in terms of aberrant biochemical processes, or 'a broken brain' – and they are confident of their advances. In Torrey's words (2001): 'Schizophrenia is firmly and unequivocally established to be a brain disease, just as surely as multiple sclerosis, Parkinson's disease, and Alzheimer's are established as brain diseases' (p. 152).

Torrey and others who make such claims are not without compelling evidence. First, some studies show that the development of schizophrenia is linked to an inherited vulnerability, i.e. to genes. First-degree relatives of people with schizophrenia appear to be three to seven times more likely to develop the disorder than people with no such relatives. Moreover, when one identical or monozygotic twin has schizophrenia, the likelihood that the other will also have schizophrenia is substantially greater. So too if one from a pair of non-identical or dizygotic twins has schizophrenia, although here the increase of incidence is not as dramatic (Gottesman, 1991). Importantly, these rates appear to be consistent when identical and non-identical twins have been adopted and raised by different families (Kety, 1987).

In addition to the links between genetics and occurrence rates, others have studied the brains of those suffering from schizophrenia, whether through post-mortem exams or computerized tomography and magnetic resonance imaging. These inquiries have found with reasonable consistency that the brains of people with schizophrenia differ in several significant ways from the brains of those without mental illness. First, and most consistently, the brains of those with schizophrenia appear to be smaller, that is, they have less overall volume and larger ventricles, the pockets within the brain which contain cerebral spinal fluid (Chua and McKenna, 1995). Research seeking to determine whether these reductions are the result of lesions or simply reductions in the size of specific regions have produced inconsistent results. Nevertheless, across these studies there is evidence that some, though not all people with schizophrenia undergo reductions in the size of (a) the superior temporal gyrus, a structure linked with the processing of auditory sensations, (b) the hippocampus, which is implicated in memory, (c) the thalamus, which is thought to play a central role in communication within the brain, and (d) the prefrontal cortex, which is associated with the ability to think in a flexible and abstract manner (e.g. Andreasen *et al.*, 1994; Breier, Buchanan, Elkashef, Munson and Gellad, 1992; Nelson, Saykin, Flashman and Riordan, 1998; Zakzanis and Heinrichs, 1999).

Other researchers have examined the brains of those suffering from schizophrenia at the level of multilayered cellular organization, or cytoarchitecture. As summarized by Heinrichs (2001), these studies have consistently found significant disarray in the organization of cells (in contrast to the brains of those without severe mental illness). With such defects in basic structural organization, effective communication among different parts of the brain may be undermined. It is possible, for instance, that individual brain cells in schizophrenia may not be in the optimal place to communicate efficiently with other brain cells, leading to insufficient coordination throughout the brain. Of note, people with schizophrenia, on average, have less gray matter than people without mental illness, that is, brain cell nuclei. While it's not clear what is happening on the cellular level, the best evidence suggests that although the number of brain cells may be similar, the amount of synaptic material has diminished.

Beyond studies of brain structures and cells, others have examined the biology of schizophrenia through behavioral or electrophysiological measures of brain activities. For example, people with schizophrenia routinely have difficulty smoothly following visual objects, which may suggest a biologically based failure to coordinate sensory input with motor behavior (Clementz and Sweeney, 1990). Irregularities in EEG (electroencephalograph) readings of people with schizophrenia also commonly appear. Some of this research suggests that people with schizophrenia show an unusual inability to synchronize brain activity with sensory input. When listening to a rhythmic tone or series of clicks, the EEG from a healthy brain synchronizes with the frequency of the tones or clicks. Research suggests that this may not occur in people with schizophrenia (Brenner, Sporns, Lysaker and O'Donnell, 2003).

With findings similar to EEG-based assessments of brain function, some research, with the aid of neuropsychological tests, has explored cognitive abilities among those suffering from schizophrenia in relation to brain function. These studies suggest that many with schizophrenia experience grave deficits in their ability to pay attention, recall, and recognize verbal and visual stimuli, again relative to the capacities of people without mental illness (Braff, 1993; Saykin et al., 1991). One popularly used test of neurocognition, the Wisconsin Card Sorting Test, requires participants to uncover rules that enable them to correctly match cards from one deck to another. Participants match cards one at a time, and each time, they are told only whether they are correct or not. Over time, they need to discover the rule according to which matches are determined. After the participant has answered correctly several times in a row, the examiner, without warning, changes the matching rules for scoring and now tells the participant they are correct if they match based on another card characteristic. Not only do people with schizophrenia have difficulties with this task when the rules change unexpectedly, but the worse they are at tracking these shifts, the more likely they are to be hospitalized more frequently and the less likely they are to be aware of the depths of their own challenges (Lysaker, Bell, Bioty and Zito, 1996; Lysaker, Bryson, Lancaster, Evans and Bell, 2003).

The view that schizophrenia reflects an aberrant biology or 'broken brain' has grown hand in hand with several developmental accounts of this condition. Stated most generally, these theories suggest that genetic vulnerability is the condition's principal ingredient, although it is not always sufficient to produce onset. Because no single gene or genetic site for such vulnerability has been found, the reigning hypothesis, often called the 'stress-diathesis' model of schizophrenia (Zubin and Spring, 1977), is that schizophrenia, like most complex behavioral phenomena, develops when there are abnormalities in a number of brain functions linked with genetic vulnerability and sufficient amounts of stress.

A leader among these developmental arguments is often called 'neurodevelopment theory' (Green, 2001). It suggests that schizo-phrenia has its roots in improper *in utero* brain development. For exam-ple, it has been hypothesized that schizophrenia may reflect a failure of cellular migration, which involves the orderly growth of brain cells during the second trimester. As a result of genetic risk and a significant stressor experienced by the mother, the fetus's brain cells pre-sumably fail to move or grow into places in the brain where they would be able to form optimal connections with other brain cells. (Note that this theory complements the findings noted above regarding disorgan-ized brain cells among those suffering from schizophrenia.) Is there evi-dence that maternal stress is linked to the development of schizophrenia? One study, conducted by Huttunen and Niskanen (1978), answers affir-matively. As described by Green (2001), this study sought to determine who was more likely to develop schizophrenia: either Finnish children under the age of 1 who lost their fathers during the Second World War, or fetuses *in utero* who suffered the same fate. Results suggested that people who were *in utero* were placed at greater risk by these stresses, perhaps indicating that *in utero* stresses for genetically vulnerable individuals may lead to higher rates of schizophrenia. War and natural catastrophes are not the only courses of stress that might interact with babies *in utero*, however. Other risk factors may include exposure to viruses such as influenza that trigger destructive antibodies (Mednick, Machon, Huttunen and Bonnet, 1988; Torrey, Bowler, Rawlings and Terrazas, 1993), malnutrition (Susser and Lin, 1992), obstetric complications (Kendell, McInneny, Juszcak and Bain, 2000), and others stressors linked to poverty and urban living (van Os, Hanssen, Bijl and Vollebergh, 2001).

A related view that does not necessarily contradict the neurodevelopmental perspective is the theory of neurodegeneration. Like Kraeplin, proponents of this view argue that people suffering from schizophrenia experience steady degradation and loss of brain function over the course of their illness. On this view, not only do the brains of people with schizophrenia fail to develop optimally, but, at some point, they show a rapid deterioration in function. This deterioration in function may be associated with alterations in the brain's structure and neurophysiological responses. Some have hypothesized, for instance, that among vulnerable individuals, either too many or too few brain cells are destroyed during early adolescent periods in which excess or under-utilized brain cells naturally die off (McGlashan and Hoffman, 2000). Studies of those who do not seek pharmacological treatment have also suggested that, for a period of up to two years after onset, significant losses in the ability to attend, remember and think flexibly may occur, which are presumably linked to the onset of some brain pathology brought about by the destruction of brain cells over a limited period of time (McGlashan, 1998). Yet another suggestion claims that neurotoxic amino acids are released within the brain during periods of symptom exacerbation and that these amino acids actively destroy brain cells (Olney and Farber, 1995). Finally, another view proposes that some who suffer from schizophrenia experience progressive brain deterioration for more than the first few years after onset such that (a) the brain continues to lose volume after the illness has begun (Delisi, Sakuma, Tew, Kushner, Hoff and Grimson, 1997), and (b) continuing and unexpectedly steep cognitive declines may occur as these men and women grow older (Bowie *et al.*, 2005; Fucetola *et al.*, 2000).

The impact of unjust social processes

Alongside the view that schizophrenia reflects a 'broken brain', there is a parallel and rich tradition of theories that regard the difficulties of schizophrenia as the byproduct of destructive social and cultural processes. For more than 200 years, various religious and reform movements have proposed that the difficulties faced by those in asylums are rooted in social rejection and inequities, as well as the neglect, if not disastrous mistreatment, which patients have encountered in hospitals. Among these movements, one finds those detailed by Whitaker (2002), which, in Europe and the United States, actively sought to remove people from asylums and mainstream society in order to promote health and self-reliance through humane interactions and work. It is worth noting that these movements continue to exist and report success (Hoffman and Kupper, 2002; Mosher, 1999). Stated most directly, in this view disability in schizophrenia is in part a reflection of medical and other forms of inhumanity. Disability and dysfunction proceed from having been shunned and denied access to needed opportunities and networks of support.

Some of the inhumane medical practices thought to cause disability have disappeared over the last half century. Since the 1950s, overtly sadistic treatment practices such as lobotomy and insulin-induced coma, which directly inflicts brain damage, have vanished. Contemporary surveys of people with schizophrenia suggest that many have found mental health professionals respectful and reliable (Coursey, Keller and Farrell, 1995). Nevertheless, broad population surveys suggest that the general public continues to hold stereotyped beliefs about severe mental illness (Swindle, Heller, Pescosolido and Kikuzawa, 2000). Categorically referred to as stigma, these stereotypes include expectations that people with schizophrenia are more likely to be violent and to behave in a generally aggressive, disorderly and impulsive manner. One also encounters opinions that people with schizophrenia cannot sustain gainful employment and are not able to reliably make informed decisions about their own welfare (Link, Phelan, Bresnahan, Stueve and Pescosolido, 1999; Pescosolido, Monahan, Link, Stueve and Kikuzawa, 1999; Phelan, Link, Stueve and Pescosolido, 2000).

Distressingly, stigma is evident across society, transcending racial and socioeconomic barriers. Across many cultures, it can be observed in the speech and behavior of community members, mental health professionals, family members, educators, employers, law enforcement officials, as well as in the media and entertainment industry (Corrigan and Penn, 1999; Lee, Lee, Chiu and Kleinman, 2005; Wahl 1999). In order to underscore the prevalence of stigma, a man with schizophrenia whom we know noted how crime stories on television sometimes end with the phrase: 'and he/she was taking antidepressants'. He then asked whether we could imagine an affirmative television news story that ended with the phrase 'and s/he was being prescribed anti-depressants.' Could there be, he inquired, news stories that observed and celebrated the achievements of people suffering from mental illness? This point is well taken.

Research suggests that stigma is more than a matter of unjustified beliefs that can prove hurtful. It often interferes with the ability of mentally ill people to meet basic needs (Link, Frances, Struening, Shrout and Dohrenwend, 1989; Wahl and Harmon, 1989). It is widely reported that stigma interferes with finding and keeping work (Bordieri and Drehmer, 1986; Link, 1987), housing (Page, 1983) and/or negotiating the legal system (Sosowsky, 1980). Research also suggests that those who hold biased beliefs towards people with severe mental illness also report a tendency to avoid or seek social distance from people they perceive as having severe mental illness (Martin, Pescosolido and Tuch, 2000). They may be tentative about socially approaching or engaging people with mental illness. In short, stigma seems to reinforce the isolation of the mentally ill, serving as a barrier to equal exchange with society at large, social services, work, and family.

Goffman (1963) has suggested that embedded in stigma is a darker and more destructive conviction, namely, that people with mental illness are less valuable than other human beings. From the perspective of the people with schizophrenia, stigma may thus leave them feeling as if they deserve their malady and/or isolation. Moreover, these beliefs may be internalized, thus effecting even more personal difficulties (Ritsher, Otilingam and Grajales, 2003; Thompson, 1988; Warner, Taylor, Powers and Hyman, 1989). For example, with sufficient exposure to stigma, persons might come to believe that they are dangerous or cannot manage their own life. As a result, they may give up and care for themselves less actively. In a recent therapy session, a young college student sought permission to get a pencil from his pocket. When asked why he needed permission, he said that he was worried the therapist (PL) would be scared. When challenged about this, he said: 'Maybe you don't think we can be trusted.' 'You mean young guys with pencils?' The patient laughed and shook his finger: 'No, you know; I'm a schizophrenic.' Not surprisingly, research confirms that experiences of stigma are associated with demoralization, depressed mood and decreased life satisfaction (Dickerson, Sommerville, Origoni, Ringel and Parente, 2002; Markowitz, 1998; Mechanic, McAlpine, Rosenfield and Davis, 1994; Rosenfield, 1997). In a two-year longitudinal study of stigma and self-concept, Wright and colleagues (2000) found that stigma, beyond producing general stress, slowly degrades a person's sense of mastery and control over their lives, and as exposure to stigma mounted, people felt less able to manage their own lives.

Just as stigma can be thought of as a force that contributes to and causes the dysfunction seen in schizophrenia, there is growing evidence that there are other destructive social forces that play a role in the development and persistence of schizophrenia. Specifically, violence and victimization may be a significant contributor to the course if not the development of the illness (Read, Perry, Moskowitz and Connolly, 2001). In one of the largest studies to date, over 700 people with varying forms of severe mental illnesses (approximately 65 percent of whom met the criteria for a schizophrenia spectrum disorder) were surveyed and asked whether they had ever experienced incidents of sexual and/or physical assault (Mueser et al., 2003). Physical and sexual victimization, in both childhood and adulthood, occurred far more often for this population than for of the general public. Particularly important was the high percentage of people who reported experiencing childhood sexual abuse. Twenty-nine percent of the men and forty-nine percent of the women surveyed reported they had been victims of childhood sexual abuse. Other studies examining smaller samples have found very similar rates in addition to correlations between the presence of childhood sexual abuse and more severe levels of hallucinations and delusions, as well as poorer psychosocial function (Lysaker, Meyer, Evans, Clements and Marks, 2001; Ross, Anderson and Clark, 1994). In a recent analysis of men with schizophrenia who were enrolled in rehabilitation, we found that a history of childhood sexual abuse predicted poorer participation in a job placement, as well as hallucinations and anxieties that were more severe and erratic (Lysaker, Beattie, Strasburger and Davis, 2005). People with schizophrenia and abuse histories dropped out of their work placements more quickly than those with schizophrenia and no abuse history. They also consistently experienced more severe levels of hallucinations and anxiety as assessed every other week during a 4-month period.

Others researchers have inquired into the living conditions experienced during childhood by people with schizophrenia. For example, Holowka and colleagues (2003) found in their small sample that nearly one out of two people diagnosed with schizophrenia reported physical neglect during their formative years, and nearly three out of four reported emotional neglect in childhood. Other research has suggested that generally disadvantageous community conditions, particularly among urban centers, could represent a risk factor for schizophrenia. Mortensen and colleagues (1999), drawing from the Civil Registration System in Denmark, used data from 1.75 million people whose mothers were born in Denmark between 1935 and 1978. This data was linked to the Danish Psychiatric Central Register, which contains records of treatment and diagnoses. From the initial group, 2669 cases of schizophrenia were identified. Based on their analyses of the correlates for people who had and did not have schizophrenia, the authors concluded that being born in a Danish urban setting was an even greater risk factor for schizophrenia than having a family history of schizophrenia. Similar research has focused on more specific elements of urbanization and their possible relation to mental illness. In these studies, one finds some links between phenomena such as poverty and racism to the development of schizophrenia (Bhugra, 2000; Mallett, Leff, Bhugra, Pang and Zhao, 2002).

Conclusion

Thus far we have outlined the wide range of symptoms and deficits that characterize the spectrum of phenomena gathered under the title 'schizophrenia'. We have also presented, in survey fashion, two central empirical explanations for the appearance of these phenomena. One regards schizophrenia as the result of abnormal biological forces derailing the lives of individuals. The other finds unjust social forces responsible for the unsettling of so many minds and lives. Schizophrenia thus presents itself to the general reader as a tidal wave propelled on the one hand by the likes of poverty, racism and childhood abuse, and on the other by disastrous declines in brain function. Or, as many have suggested, perhaps both fault lines interact (Carter and Flesher, 1995; Walker and Diforio, 1997).

While much of the research we have cited strikes us as valid by current scientific standards, we are nevertheless led to ask about the subject tossed about on this sea of biological and social forces. The clients whose stories we have alluded to above experienced periods when they loved, worked and dreamt. They had lives that once seemed full and orderly. Yet each now faces an uncertain future. How should we conceive of these lives as they live them? There is a metaphorical suggestiveness to talk of people washed out to sea, but such images do not, as Barham (1993) has suggested, succeed in 'characterizing adequately … just what … is humanly the case in schizophrenic predicaments' (p. 79). The image fails because it only offers us an object beset by forces, not the person undergoing them, that is, experiencing him or herself beset by and scrambling for a life amid those forces.

Let us be more precise. Can thoroughly third-person approaches to schizophrenia adequately grasp the phenomenon, or is there an ineliminable first-person dimension to the illness? The perspectives we have reviewed in this first chapter are quintessential third-person accounts. Like all empirical lines of inquiry, they analyze human lives as nexuses of causal forces, and with an eye on interactions that produce effects characteristic of schizophrenia. To be sure, we acknowledge and respect the explanatory power of these accounts and the therapies they enable and continue to refine. But in principle, they exclude the experience of symptoms as phenomena that one undergoes, and not just as a perceiver. Schizophrenia interrupts the lives of people struggling to find and create security and meaning in a world of contingency. From this perspective, that of an agent, symptoms are added contingencies, that is, threats to human well-being that must be interpreted and constructively engaged. We lose this facet of the phenomenon if we do not consider what it is like to live with phenomena like delusions, hallucinations, disordered cognitions, stigmatization, and/or loss of affect. Third-person views thus risk 'amputating madness from the man who embodies it', to recall the words of Stanghellini (2004, p. 46). Brain cells accumulating or dying off are not the subjects of a life, but those suffering from schizophrenia are, and it is in the context of such a life that some basic facets of schizophrenia lie, or so we shall argue.

However, the issue is not simply one of descriptive fidelity. Working exclusively within third-person perspectives may lead us to see people as passive beings locked in faulty bodies or faulty social networks. If a goal of therapy is to empower another's agency, then we may very well need to consider their travails from the standpoint of an agent. As Barnham notes, 'a particular merit' of 'taking the schizophrenic person seriously ... as an active participant in social life' is that it may allow us 'to identify more adequately where (at points) he fails as a social agent' (1993, p. 78). Said otherwise, we may need to preserve the first-person in the study of schizophrenia in order to understand what has changed and, most importantly, what can change in lives profoundly interrupted by schizophrenia. But how should we go about locating the first-person and its agency amidst schizophrenia?

Chapter 2

Sense of self in schizophrenia

At the end of Chapter 1, we suggested that even the most thorough third-person accounts fail to fully portray the phenomenon of schizophrenia. Not that objective symptoms, cortical dysfunction, neurocognitive compromise, or social injustice are of marginal interest for the study of schizophrenia. Rather, any explanation which ignores the first-person dimensions of the illness limits our understanding of it and, perhaps, our ability to treat it. While we will refine our conception of the first-person in Chapter 3, for now, the concept stands to remind us that human beings are creatures who experience events even as they strive to respond productively to those events. Our claim, then, is that alongside symptoms and their causes, one must track and engage *sense of self* among those with schizophrenia, for its fate is integral to the illness.

Exploring sense of self

Admittedly, 'sense of self' is a slippery phrase. It has the danger of suggesting many indefinite things. For our immediate purposes, we wish for it to indicate how one's being is disclosed to oneself, say as female, a citizen of Nigeria, generous, and a doctor. It is how we are experienced by ourselves. What is sensed in a 'sense of self' is the character and welfare of one's being, and it is given in a more or less integrated series, or in the form of a 'life'. In the language of Hegel (1807/1979), sense of self involves a way in which our being is *for* us, that is, available for interpretation and action. In this idiom, we could say that our qualities and traits, what Hegel would regard as our being *in*-itself, are disclosed to us as matters to be reckoned with and engaged. For example, should one appear to oneself as 'white', that will reflect a certain historical fate with certain historical prospects, and not simply some morphological trait, and so too with being short or tall, a banker or day laborer, a U.S. citizen or one of the nationless Roma. We could thus say that 'sense of self' indicates how one finds oneself, as in the English idiom, 'how did you find the Oregon coast?' to which one might say, 'rocky, magnificent, difficult going, windy, a great place for meditation, rugged, sublime'.

Finding oneself in the manner noted above names a way in which our being is disclosed to itself in the project of its life. This merits underscoring. On our interpretation, 'sense of self' involves what Heidegger terms a *Haltung* (1929/1993), a practical orientation or posture towards the vicissitudes of a life taken up and undergone by the one who lives that life. A 'sense of self' thus not only registers states of affairs, such as qualities and traits, but also, and from the outset, their significance for one or more life projects.

'Sense of self' is not only a slippery phrase, but also an elusive phenomenon if one adopts the vocabulary and methodology of much contemporary experimental science. If one does not begin within the context of a life, of a being unfolding through its ongoing interpretations of and responses to its fate, sense of self will appear, as it might have to Hume, as an idea in search of an object. In order to track sense of self therefore, one has to see a person as more than a nexus of causal forces, and schizophrenia as more than a set of symptoms for which causal origins must be found. Rather, one must also regard symptoms as phenomena undergone by an interpretive, purposive being.[1]

Interestingly, clinical contexts may also obscure a client's sense of self. Most research regards the participant as a patient receiving (or rejecting) treatment, and thus as someone with something wrong that could be healed if only it were properly understood. If the patient has voluntarily sought treatment, they have likely done so with the expectation that some professional could discern what was wrong and how to help. If they have entered treatment involuntarily, that is, if they have been committed against their will, it is because someone else, possibly a relative in conjunction with the courts, has analogously decided that their troubles will be better understood and treated by health care professionals. In both cases, a third-person perspective overdetermines the phenomena at hand.

Consider what often happens in a clinic. 'What has brought you here?' 'What seems to be the trouble?' These are common, opening questions. Formal research begins in a similar manner. 'Do you think you have a mental illness and if so what is it?' 'What symptoms do you have?' 'Have you felt sad or blue?' 'Do you have the experience of feeling especially famous or important?' 'Have you had the experience of seeing or hearing things others do not hear or see?' These are common elements of established, semi-structured interviews. The patients or clients may feel, therefore, that their role is to offer a concrete symptom or difficulty that could be treated or rated. In a research interview, a patient might say, for example: 'I hear voices from God urging me to run in the marathon on Saturday.' The interviewer might then explore how often and when the voice is heard. Our suggestion is not that these are improper or unhelpful questions. We suggest only that within such contexts, first-person accounts of schizophrenia are rarely ventured or solicited. Instead, the participant is encouraged to and often does present atomized symptoms. It would seem, then, that in many if not most clinical settings, the categories of appraisal derive from the third-person perspective of the mental health profession.

Here is a more concrete instance of the inadvertent, methodological limits at work in clinical settings. It is drawn from a conversation with a man suffering from schizophrenia. The conversation, conducted during the 1990s, occurred during an unpublished research interview, whose purpose was to understand beliefs about and reactions to auditory hallucinations. The man, who was in his thirties, from an upper-middle class family, appeared eager to participate. In answer to the first few questions, he indicated that he heard voices tell him to run in an upcoming marathon. We asked: 'Do you find them distressing?' 'Absolutely,' he replied. We asked: 'Do you wish it would stop?' He again was unambiguously affirmative. 'Why do you wish it would stop?' Here he laughed, and with a look of amusement, explained: 'It would certainly make my psychiatrist feel accomplished.'

Here we are reminded that even in clinical settings, one inadvertently can look past both what someone is experiencing and how they are responding to those experiences. In doing so, one 'amputates', in the words of Stenghellini, the person from the disorder. We assert that this also amputates human beings from their life, at least as it is given to them as theirs, and, once removed from the context of their life as it is disclosed to them in the course of their lives, their experience becomes a matter for others to understand. In order to avoid these excisions, one needs to keep an eye on someone's own experience of schizophrenia, including his or her interpretation of and response to those experiences. Said another way, in order to access sense of self amid schizophrenia, one needs to return the illness to the life it has disrupted.

A history of reflection on first-person experience in schizophrenia

While the majority of the literature concerning schizophrenia seeks an ever more complete third-person account, it would be inaccurate to say that no one has considered the experiences of those with schizophrenia. As we will document, people from widely divergent traditions, while addressing various clinical, psychological, and social issues have explored what it is like to live with schizophrenia. In strikingly similar ways, many have suggested that from the first-person perspective, schizophrenia often involves a fundamental alteration in self-experience or sense of self. Moreover, that alteration involves a sense of oneself as significantly less vital than one had been previously.

In what follows, we will present an overview of these observations. In particular we will detail descriptions of the disruption of self-experience in schizophrenia from the schools of traditional psychiatry, existential psychiatry, psychoanalysis, psychosocial rehabilitation and phenomenology. We will then develop some questions raised by these observations in order to articulate our task concretely, namely, the development of a comprehensive, first-person account of sense of self in schizophrenia, one which neither amputates the person from the disorder, nor denies or loses sight of the social and biological realities involved in the genesis and course of schizophrenia.

Traditional psychiatry

While Bleuler and Kraeplin cataloged schizophrenia's many manifestations, each noted how the condition also compromised sense of self.

After providing a lengthy apology and explanation for his decision to create the term 'schizophrenia', Bleuler, in a section labeled 'The definition of the disease', observes: 'If disease is marked the personality loses its unity ... one set of complexes dominates the personality for a time, while other groups of ideas or drives are "split off" and seem either partially or completely impotent' (1911/1950, p. 9). Later, discussing what he called accessory symptoms (e.g. hallucinations, delusions and memory disturbance), he adds:

> Everything may seem different; one's own person as well as the external world ... in a completely unclear manner *so that the patient hardly knows how to orient himself either inwardly or outwardly* ... The person 'loses his boundaries in time and space'.
>
> (p. 143 – italics added)

Kraeplin devotes far less time to this problem, and yet he presumes that the destruction of the self is constitutive of the disorder. For instance, he notes in the first sentence of his 1919 (2002) considerations: 'Dementia praecox consists of a series of states, the common characteristic of which is a peculiar destruction of the internal connection of the psychic personality' (p. 3). Moreover, given its focus on what such people can no longer do or even hope to do, his work can be read as a portrait of a ruined subject.

Beyond these classical observations, one finds another medically oriented psychiatrist, Schneider, who, 50 years later, also catalogued the disturbances of schizophrenia. While Bleuler focused on disturbances of thinking, and Kraelpin upon losses of interest and affect, Schneider's principal concerns were bizarre delusions and hallucinations (Koehler, Guth and Grimm, 1977). Nevertheless, he also, at least indirectly, spoke about schizophrenia in terms of disturbed self-experience, noting how delusions and hallucinations leave one unable to distinguish internal and external events, thus severely undermining interpersonal relationships.

What this brief review shows is that without thematizing the phenomenon of sense of self, classical psychiatry nevertheless observes how schizophrenia often involves profoundly disorganized and unstable psyches, and that such disturbances lead to skewed and difficult relations with oneself and others. Such phenomena are still observed from the third-person, however, as if the people in question were poorly running engines. Yet the substance of these observations is echoed in the years to come, and it does show some feel for the life terrain upon which sense of self arises within schizophrenia.

Existential psychiatry

Seventy years later, R. D. Laing (1978) contested the biological interpretation of schizophrenia, and called for a radically existential recasting of notions regarding madness. Despite his opposition to many of the tenants of traditional psychiatry, his observations in *The Divided Self* are similar to Blueler, Kraeplin and Schneider's, although he argued that subjective disturbance informs the essence of schizophrenia. On his view, someone with schizophrenia is fundamentally alienated, and experiences 'a rent in his relation with his world … and a disruption of his relation with himself'. Such a person, according to Laing, does not and cannot feel 'together with' others or 'at home' in the world. He or she is unable to experience him or herself as 'a complete person' (p. 17). In such states, it is unclear from moment to moment who or what one is, and the boundaries of self and other seem tenuous and unreliable. Moreover, one's world is terrifying, as if it were 'liable at any moment to crash in and obliterate all identity' (p. 45).

Focusing even more intently on the psychological experience of schizophrenia, Boss suggested that schizophrenia involves the experience of an 'encroachment' on one's

> ability to be responsive and open to what is encountered … First they cannot open themselves fully to the meaningful address of what they encounter … so that they cannot respond with all their faculties to the normally accepted significance … of those things and events. Second they are unable to maintain a free stance vis-à-vis their perceptions of what they encounter.
>
> (1979, p. 235)

In view of this degree of personal destabilization, Boss regarded schizophrenia as the 'radically incomplete manifestation of the free and self-reliant selfhood that normally characterizes a human being. Therefore, schizophrenia is an illness that can be characterized only negatively' (p. 236).

Like the principal figures of classical psychiatry, Laing and Boss remarked upon the disordered nature of psychic life in the throes of schizophrenia. Boss in particular echoed the earlier sense of radical incapacity and loss, and while he presented such a self as overwhelmed, it is Laing who had a finer feeling for what it is like to be that self. It was thus Laing who begins to articulate what the sense of self amid schizophrenia might entail: alienation, incompletion, and terror. In other words, whereas Boss speaks mostly of loss and incapacity, Laing helps us to begin to see a life interpreting and responding to its own incipient dispersion.

Psychoanalysis

Psychoanalysts have also widely noted that people with schizophrenia experience and openly report a diminished sense of identity along with tenuous boundaries between self and other (Frankel, 1993; Selzer and Schwartz, 1994). As with most psychoanalytic theories, this view can be traced back to Freud, in particular to his assertion (1957) that schizophrenia occurs when one detaches from the world and internalizes one's energies to the point that all consensually valid meaning is lost. In such a state, one has removed all emotional or personal investment from the world and descended into radical narcissism.

Importantly, Freud's account implies that psychoanalytic treatment is impossible for people in this state. Radically narcissistic, and thus unable to relate sufficiently to their therapists, those suffering from schizophrenia presumably cannot learn about themselves from their unfolding relationship with an analyst. This presumption, and hence Freud's conception, became an object of significant debate within psychoanalysis as therapists began to test the notion that psychoanalysis or psychoanalytic psychotherapy was impossible when psychosis was present. Particularly in the United States, psychoanalysts tried to relate to and treat people with schizophrenia, using the clinical relationship as the basis for intervention. They reported that profound bonds quickly emerged between patient and therapist. This was noted to occur especially when the therapist was patient and open to knowing the client as more than a ruined subject. Fromm-Reichmann (1954) and Searles (1965), who treated inpatients at Chestnut Lodge, Sullivan (1962), who treated inpatients at the White Institute, and Knight (1946), who treated inpatients at the Menninger Clinic, all contended that meaningful relations with people with schizophrenia emerged in therapy. Not only did they find that their patients were able to form intimate bonds, but also that their mental health improved as these bonds developed.

What intrigues us about this development is the turn towards psychotherapy with people suffering from schizophrenia. Clinicians were conversing with institutionalized people suffering from schizophrenia as often as five times per week, week after week, and really, only listening. On the basis of such work, Fromm-Reichman and others came to describe how schizophrenia involved both a profoundly fractured sense of identity and enormous longing for closeness. The problem was, even though occasional connections were possible, sustained engagements were difficult, and clients often became quite anxious even in brief engagements. The suggestion, then, was that in the thick of schizophrenia, closeness with others was longed for, but also a source of enormous terror and fear. Frosh suggested (1983) that when engaging others, people with schizophrenia experience themselves as on the verge of either disintegration or contraction to a bare awareness of nothingness. On this view, then, schizophrenia involves a sense of oneself as either too weak or insufficiently structured to survive being in the world with others.

From another angle, one somewhat reminiscent of Bleuer's observations, other treating analysts have observed that intrapsychic relations can also appear threatening to those suffering from schizophrenia (Bak, 1954; Bion, 1967). For instance, if strong feelings of guilt or aggression entered into awareness, terror ensued. According to these observations, in schizophrenia the self is experienced as unable to interpret and engage the full rage of its fate effectively.

Like Laing, psychoanalytic treatments of schizophrenia evidence a good feel for the illness's first-person dimensions. Once again we find a self that experiences itself as anxiety ridden in the face of others, although here, we also find a self that experiences itself as unequal to the task of containing its own affects. Psychoanalytic literature thus offers us a rather rich picture of the sense of self that is characteristic of schizophrenia, namely: (1) a self longing for connection with others, but simultaneously terrified of social encounters, and (2) a self too weak to successfully respond to life, particularly when experiences prove provocative and demanding.

Psychosocial rehabilitation research

In the recent history of psychiatric treatment, it has been widely observed that as psychoanalysis lost its vanguard status, psychosocial rehabilitation rapidly became the most researched and recommended form of non-pharmacological treatment of schizophrenia. In general, psychosocial rehabilitation entails a wide range of transtheoretical interventions, such as supported employment and social skills training. Oriented towards skill and function enhancement, it considers how people can develop and pursue personally meaningful goals, and how they might live reasonably full lives. Among its research projects, one finds several longitudinal studies of recovery processes (Strauss, Hafez, Lieberman and Harding, 1985), that consider multidimensional outcomes as well as the personal and social context in which illness and recovery occurs (Davidson, 2003).

Given its desire to deepen the personal meaning of those who suffer from it, we are unsurprised that schizophrenia's first-person facets have received sustained attention in psychosocial rehabilitation research. Some studies present people who fail to fit into their worlds, and who manifest enormous desire for closeness as well as deep sensitivity to rejection (Davidson and Stayner, 1997). Others contain multiple references to people who experience little sense of agency, and who struggle to distinguish themselves from their illness (Estroff, 1989; Roe and Ben-Yishai, 1999; Young and Ensign, 1999; Williams and Collins, 1999). Painted in a uniquely longitudinal light, these studies offer portraits of people who, in the midst of their disorder, feel eclipsed by their illness. They may reach the point where it seems as if they are nothing more than an amorphous disturbance, something akin to the ruined subject noted above.

Thinking generally about these and similar phenomena, Davidson (2003) suggests that the experience of severe mental illness, and presumably, schizophrenia in particular, does not merely involve alienation and uncertainty, but also a loss of authority with regard to one's own sense of oneself. Such people, he writes, may have stopped seeing themselves as 'somebody, somewhere about whom a story might be told' (p. 211). As a result, they risk living a life in which they are invisible to themselves as protagonists (Roe and Davidson, 2005). The rehabilitation literature contains another observation worth reporting. It suggests that people suffering from schizophrenia can recover a more empowered sense of self through the active construction of narratives regarding both their illness (Roe and Kravetz, 2003) and their relation to it (Roe and Ben Yishai, 1999), if those constructions are enhanced by ongoing interactions and engagement with the environment (Roe, 2001). Psychoanalysis also allows for recovery from schizophrenia, but only on the basis of interventions from analysts who have privileged knowledge. In contrast, Roe and his colleagues, as well as Davidson, find that people with schizophrenia can recover a sense of self as a matter of course, and at their own direction. Along the way, these authors also remind us of the essential role of first-person narratives in the elaboration of sense of self. They claim that people with schizophrenia, along with the rest of humanity, constantly construct stories that contextualize how we find ourselves, that is, how we interpret personal welfare.

While echoing previous observations regarding the alienation and longing that characterize schizophrenia, psychosocial rehabilitation research seems to do so with the first-person more firmly in mind. Moreover, these theorists thicken the first-person experience with an explicit narrative dimension, which proves instrumental to their conceptualization of recovery. By offering insights into selves flummoxed by their own felt lack of agency, these studies further concretize the diminished selfhood observed by so many others.

Phenomenology

With strong links to German and French philosophy and psychiatry, another group of theorists has studied how consciousness is structured in schizophrenia. For example, the French psychiatrist, Minkowski (1927/1987), suggested that schizophrenia involves a loss of 'vital contact with reality'. Looking at the first-person experience of this loss, he found a lack of ongoing, temporal synthesis, which leaves one without enough integrated experience to sustain a sense of self. The result is that one loses touch with the 'moving stream which envelops us at all points and constitutes the milieu without which [one does not] know how to live' (p. 191). One thus might say of the person with schizophrenia that 'although he knows where he is, he does not feel as if he is in that place … the term 'I exist' has no real meaning for him' (p. 196).

Since Minkowski, phenomenological approaches to schizophrenia have more or less revolved around the work of Blankenburg (2001), a German psychiatrist inspired by philosophers Husserl and Heidegger, and the Swiss psychiatrist, Binswanger (cf. Mishara, 1997). Blankenburg argued that schizophrenia renders self and world incomprehensible, because it fundamentally undermines what he terms 'common sense', a prereflective capacity to gauge what any given situation demands. For example, one might be unable to order possible interpretations along the line of how probable they are, as in the case of paranoia. Or, one may lose a feel for social mores and the like. Blankenburg writes:

> What becomes striking for those around the patient is that there is a withering away of a sense of tact, a feeling for the proper thing to do in situations, a loss of awareness of the current fashions … a general indifference towards what might be disturbing to others.

> (p. 306)

Or, to offer a third variant, one might fail to find continuity in things and events. In the words of Schwartz and colleagues:

> If one inhabits a world in which the causal relations among objects and even the continuous identity of objects themselves is uncertain, unreliable and shifting, then it is difficult to speak to others in a way that would make sense.

> (2005, p. 112)

Extending this logic, Stanghellini (2004) suggests that a loss of pre-reflectively operative common sense would fundamentally disrupt self-experience in the context of relatedness. On this view, the problem becomes one of rote or stagnant interpretations of situations.

Without a living connection to the world, one that establishes a dialogue between desire and the world's feedback, psychosocial dysfunction becomes less a lack of social skills than 'a defective dialectic between the two poles of the self: the individual characteristics embodied by the "I" and the social demands embodied by the "me"' (p. 78). Moreover, in the wake of these disconnects, made evident in failed social exchanges, Stanghellini notes that people with schizophrenia are forced to confront the poverty of their grasp of things, which leaves them suspended in a 'nothingness' that most of us are protected from by the adequate grasp of the world that common sense provides.

In a recent paper, Mishara (2004) considers two ways of explaining the loss of common sense. The first of these he categorizes as 'Apollonian', following Nietzsche's dichotomy of personality types. The Apollonian view comprises a range of arguments, which suggest that common sense withers under an inward gaze of radical intensity. Perhaps the most popular proponent of this view is Louis Sass (1992). He argues that despite a variety of manifestations, schizophrenia, at its core, involves 'hyperreflexive' people. On his view, people with schizophrenia are self-aware to an extreme degree. This results in their feeling like an object, alienated from the world, and devitalized. Analyzed to death, one's spontaneity dries up, and one's basic grasp of life fragments into tenuously related elements, including one's own first-person perspective on the world. From this perspective, one might say, therefore, that schizophrenia is a matter of too much rather than too little self-experience.

In contrast to Apollonian views, like Sass's, Mishara considers an alternative, which he labels 'Dionysian', whose roots lie in Blankenburg and Binswanger. On the Dionysian view, common sense fails because perceptual and automatic meaning processing are disrupted 'from below'. For example, probabilistic reasoning may suffer due to fundamental brain dysfunctions (Mishara, 2001; 2004). Common sense is thereby undermined, because one is unable to successfully apprehend a world of embodied feelings and thought that others simultaneously share, and to the point that, over time, one no longer trusts one's grasp of things.[2]

Mishara (2004; 2005) has also suggested that such disturbances involve disruptions in pre-reflectively operative bodily experience, which produce an '*inability to shift awareness from its current focus to potentially relevant information in the background*' (p. 144 – emphasis in the original). The result includes a sense of oneself as befuddled by and even disconnected from one's ongoing bodily negotiations of the world. If Mishara is right, then schizophrenia is less a matter of excessive analysis than the pre-reflective dispersion of whatever fields of meaning one might hope to analyze. The meaning of the world is beyond analysis because of disruptions that occur at the moment when the subject apprehends the world.

When set alongside its predecessors and rivals, phenomenological analyses of schizophrenia, particularly with regard to sense of self, distinguish themselves with their structural focus on the disorder's first-person dimensions. They observe anxiety, feelings of emptiness, and disordered psyches, but also tie these phenomena to breakdowns in perceptual capacities, what many call common sense. This is of particular interest because it suggests that sense of self is less a matter of introspection than a phenomenon that accompanies, perhaps even arises out of worldly engagements.

Looming questions

Among the range of perspectives we've considered, a general sense of self, as it occurs in schizophrenia, is coalescing. First, it is mistaken to regard schizophrenia as an utter collapse of self or the retreat of a person into complete self-referentiality. Instead, people suffering from schizophrenia maintain a sense of self, and therein find themselves threatened by and occasionally overwhelmed by intersubjective and powerful subjective experiences. They thus find themselves alienated from both self and other, living a life that is out of joint and at the 'edge of the common' (Barham, 1993), which often affects feelings of emptiness. Moreover, such a life appears diminished when compared with what had been the case before onset. These observations suggest, then, that alongside its range of biological and social factors, schizophrenia also involves a variety of first-person phenomena, including a widespread awareness of diminishment.

In the following chapters, we want to address how one's sense of self could fray and diminish over time. To that end, we will consider some of the first-person inflected elements and processes that seem to be compromised with the onset and development of schizophrenia. How is it that people, over the course of their illness, *find themselves* at the edge of the common, threatened by a looming, potentially overwhelming world of experiences and relations?

Now, authors from the schools of phenomenology and psychoanalysis have proposed potential answers to this question. Some have suggested, for instance, that diminishments in self are expressions of pre-existing alterations in self experience, that these alterations can be observed in early life, and that they are necessary for the development of the disorder during the tumult of adolescence and early adulthood. Some psychoanalysts, for instance, have argued that certain children do not fully internalize their early interactions with caretakers. Some basic, constitutional deficit presumably prevents some children from building their identity out of early interactions with parental figures, and this leaves them with a hollow, empty self that barely manages to exist prior to illness, and which cannot manage anxiety (Wexler, 1971). Minkowski, on the other hand, suggests that a disharmony of person and world predates the emergence of formal symptoms, that life prior to onset 'evolved in fits and starts ... not a continuous line, supple and elastic but one broken in several places' (p. 206). Bovet and Parnas (1993) argue that from an early age onwards, a basic attunement with the world is lacking in those who later face psychosis. They suggest that some failure of 'self temporalization' occurs, such that the 'subject's potential to project himself into possible future and anticipate himself is diminished' (p. 584).

While offering valid lines of inquiry, particularly when combined with biological and social analyses of the pertinent phenomena, these studies pursue directions different than our own. Our concern is not vulnerability, important as that issue is. Rather, we wish to explore how a self, vulnerable or not, begins to experience diminishment. As we will see in Chapters 5 and 6, these experiences may be relevant to vulnerability, but that is not our initial concern. Instead, the issue is how people come to sense themselves as fundamentally less than they used to be – but perhaps this remains too abstract. Let us close this chapter, therefore, by recollecting the travails of two men suffering from schizophrenia.

Illustrations

In order to think more concretely about what a diminished sense of self might mean in the context of schizophrenia, let us consider two lives affected by it. As in the case of everyone else described in this book, these lives are partly fictionalized. We say 'partly' because each case is based on Paul Lysaker's experiences with multiple people under routine and voluntary psychotherapeutic conditions. The cases, drawn from a period of over 20 years, occurred in a variety of outpatient clinics, which were located in various urban, suburban and rural areas of the United States. That said, the names and all details that might identify single individuals have been systematically changed to protect confidentiality. These materials are thus not biographical accounts of specific people.

Case Study A: Frank

Frank, whom we briefly discussed in Chapter 1, is a man first beset with symptoms around the age of 21. Because he was a psychotherapy client for over one year before his psychotic symptoms began, his case is especially revealing. In fact, initially, nothing distinguished him from anyone else who might show up in a therapist's office. He had never experienced psychosis, but wanted to discuss his uncertainty about the course his life was taking regarding love and work. He explained in a perfectly coherent manner that he was unhappy and struggling to find a place in life where he belonged. He had recently attended a prestigious college on the west coast of the United States where he had been accepted to an elite computer science program. He had barely passed his first-year classes, however. This disappointed him and his parents, who were paying full tuition, and so the family decided that he would move back home and attend a less expensive local college.

Frank had been raised by his parents and had been an average student in high school who dated regularly in adolescence. He routinely socialized with a group of close friends while growing up. He and his family had always considered him college-bound. Neither one of his parents was ever treated for a psychiatric condition, though one of his father's uncles may have suffered from psychosis. In adolescence, Frank had been in individual counseling for anxiety and panic-like symptoms and had been prescribed an anti-anxiety medication.

As the initial conversations in psychotherapy grew increasingly intimate and positively toned, and as a therapeutic relationship developed, Frank expressed frustration with his financial dependence on his parents. He spoke of shame concerning his lack of effort in school. He also wondered whether he should have broken off his relationship with a high school girlfriend and whether he should try and rekindle their romance, even though she was involved with a former friend. He talked about mourning a former music teacher who committed suicide while he was at college, and he wondered what it meant that his teacher was supposed to have ordered and eaten a pizza the night he shot himself. He was angry with his mother for being short with his father, but he also recollected times when, smelling of grease from his work as a mechanic, his father would return home and Frank would run to meet his car.

Frank was an intelligent person with a dry sense of humor, but with little sense of personal direction. He loved music and relished the hours he spent playing the trumpet. Over the first 10 months of psychotherapy, Frank appeared to gradually discover that he was quite angry with his family, and that he directed this anger towards others. He also thought that he might have even thwarted his own efforts to succeed at college as well as his relationship with the woman he sometimes thought he still loved.

After roughly a year and a half, Frank decided he knew what he had to do and decided to take a break from therapy. Two-and-a-half months later, he phoned. After an extended vacation with his family he had begun to experience acute psychosis. Seen immediately after his family contacted the clinic, he was utterly consumed with the belief that the spouse of a former teacher was arranging his assassination. He appeared frightened and argumentative. He explained in an uncharacteristically pressured manner that symbols on the backs of road signs across the state detailed particular sexual feelings that had been inserted into him, and that, at any moment, 'they could come' for him. He seemed tense and anxious during session to the point of acting as if he did not recognize his surroundings, even though he had been visiting his therapist in the same office for years.

Despite immediate pharmacological intervention, the psychosis did not remit. Six-and-a-half months later, Frank was still certain his demise might be around the corner. The trust that characterized the therapeutic relationship was gone. There were long silences, and Frank rejected attempts to understand or empathize. He finally blew up and accused the therapist of being a 'traitor'. He was furious that the therapist would not affirm the reality of the danger he faced. This meant that the therapist was no longer on his side, but an enemy. Unsure what to say, the therapist noted that Frank seemed enraged. Frank then observed, correctly, that there was anger in the therapist's voice. The therapist acknowledged his frustration, explaining that he felt that their work was hindered because they could only talk about his persecution. They not only no longer discussed Frank's love of music, his girlfriend, his music teacher etc., but it seemed as if Frank was forbidden, by himself, even to think about these things. Frank nodded, suggesting tacit agreement, and grew quiet. He finally explained that being persecuted was all he could think about, and he demanded that he and his therapist consider his obsession as a matter of necessity, not choice. Elaborating, he confessed that if he stopped thinking about his persecution, everything became unbearable. Without these thoughts, he felt only 'emptiness and nothingness', a subjective state infinitely more painful than fearing a death he might still avoid. As weeks passed and psychotherapy continued, he said that the person he once was, the person the therapist had previously known, had 'exploded'. Frank existed only as remnants kept in the general vicinity of one another by a weak and unreliable form of 'gravity'. He had lost something essential about the person he had been. Though diminished in his own eyes, he was fully aware of his loss, as were his family and therapist.

Frank's presentations of his experiences of delusions, of what it was like to have them, to live under them, evidences the presence of someone who, though in the midst of schizophrenia, can be engaged with regard to his schizophrenia. Moreover, this movement between feelings of emptiness and feelings of persecution evidences a first-person dimension to Frank's illness that demands interpretation. In fact, no understanding of his illness would be complete without it. The symptoms of schizophrenia do not belong to the one who suffers them like a color belongs to a plastic cup. Presumably, a cup does not experience itself through its being green or plastic or squat. Frank's symptoms, however, contain a reflexive dimension that is part and parcel of their occurrence; they disclose to him a sense of his own welfare in the world. (To rely again on Hegel's language, Frank's symptoms are ways in which he is for-himself). More generally, the point is that phenomena like feelings of persecution structurally entail finding oneself persecuted, which implicates an enormous range of associated phenomena, for example, 'finding oneself', some scene wherein one finds oneself, which includes persecuting agents, and so forth, and irrespective of whether one is actually being persecuted. We emphasize this because it implies that, should one fail to account for the reflexive dimension of symptoms such as someone finding him or herself persecuted, unable to commit to courses of action, or generally diminished, then one has failed to fully account for that symptom. As schizophrenia is an illness wherein human beings find themselves confronted by symptoms like delusions and/or an inability to commit to courses of action, one cannot do justice to schizophrenia unless one addresses its manifold first-person dimensions.

Like Frank, Grieg presented himself as diminished, as having been ruined at some point. He even went so far as to suggest that his life had been absorbed by mental illness. Nevertheless, he remained aware of these transformations, and thus one could engage him on these matters, on what it felt like, and how he struggled to make do. It is thus clear that for him, schizophrenia was something that he underwent. He interpreted its disenabling complexities, and he struggled to address the problems they threw in his way. So, in order to better appreciate the course that Grieg's life took, we feel compelled to explore the dimensions of these experiences and efforts.

Case Study B: Grieg

Grieg is a man who entered psychotherapy in his late forties. Like many, he had never been involved in any kind of counseling until the onset of psychosis. After his psychosis began, he was consumed by beliefs that celebrities on television were praising his masculinity, and that he had performed supernatural feats for which others would hunt him down and publicly humiliate, possibly even kill him. He also expressed significant levels of anxiety and noted feeling sad and worried most of the day, nearly every day. He spent a great deal of time alone, and expressed little interest in the thoughts or feelings of others. As we might expect from our review in Chapter 1, testing revealed grave impairments in Grieg's ability to store verbal material in memory or to think flexibly about abstract matters.

Initially, it was hard to know much if anything about Grieg's experience of schizophrenia. In conversations, he would return again and again to implausible remarks. One could thus see that he had symptoms and deficits, but who was he? As his psychotherapy progressed, Grieg reconstructed his story. He was the oldest of several children, and his mother owned a local laundromat. His parents divorced when he was nine. Neither remarried. His father worked periodically as a carpenter and his mother as an accountant. Grieg's father had suffered from psychosis and alcoholism, and his mother had an eating disorder. His father's psychosis resulted in several lengthy stays at a nearby state psychiatric hospital, an institution known locally for neglect and abuse. Later, Grieg would also be confined there.

Grieg's parents divorced while he was a child, and so he lived in several places while growing up. He first lived with his father, then with an older cousin, and finally with his mother and her new boyfriend. Grieg was an average student who dated several girls in high school. He also was involved in many extracurricular activities, including taking photographs for the school newspaper. He recalled particularly strong attachments to his father's mother and one of his younger brothers. He also noted 'blue' periods during adolescence, when he would avoid contact with others because it was hard to be around 'happy people' when there was so much trouble in his family and in his heart.

After high school, Grieg joined the military and went to basic training. As in Frank's case, he underwent a drastic change in the ensuing months. He became certain that a bomb was planted somewhere nearby. He found special messages in the newspapers, saw visions, heard the sounds of the bomb's timing mechanism through an air vent and was soon in an army hospital, receiving electroconvulsive shock treatments.

A year later, Grieg was living with his mother, working and taking medication. He found that his 'symptoms' were suddenly gone. He wrote off his experience of psychosis as 'something beyond explanation', and soon was in love and married. He and his wife had three children, and he remembered these years as 'happy'. He purchased a house and kept the same job. After four years though, he and his wife had grown distant. They worked different shifts and Grieg had started to drink more than he should. Then one of his younger brothers was killed as his car crossed the railroad tracks one morning. Grieg again started to feel himself 'go'. He heard and saw things others couldn't hear or see. The television spoke to him at length, even when turned off. He began to panic and sensed that others could read his thoughts. He withdrew, entered a hospital, and his wife divorced him. He found himself lost in a way he had not known before. He simply couldn't do what he used to do. With his mother's guidance, he was able to see his children weekly, but did little else. Often, he brought them to her house and watched television while his mother attended to them. During this time, 'I was mental illness,' he said.

Before too long, though, he again found work, this time in a nearby town. His symptoms vanished, although this time, he did not adhere to medications. He dated some, and two years later, was again in love. He lived with this woman for several years and had another child. This time though, Grieg kept losing jobs. There were days he did not leave their apartment, convinced that others were reading his mind and that there was a bomb in a local church. During this time, he again regarded himself as 'mental illness'. When asked what happened to the person he used to be, he could only shrug his shoulders and sit silently. When pushed on the issue, he eventually explained: 'That's the hell of it ... some days you just are not there.'

Like Frank, Grieg presented himself as diminished, as having been ruined at some point. He even went so far as to suggest that his life had been absorbed by mental illness. Nevertheless, he remained aware of these transformations, and thus one could engage him on these matters, on what it felt like, and how he struggled to make do. It is thus clear that for him, schizophrenia was something that he underwent. He interpreted its disenabling complexities, and he struggled to address the problems they threw in his way. So, in order to better appreciate the course that Grieg's life took, we feel compelled to explore the dimensions of these experiences and efforts.

Questions for an account of first-person perspectives in schizophrenia

The stories of both these lives illustrate people experiencing their own diminishment. According to Frank, he lost what he had been, and his paranoid delusions were all that that kept him from dissolving into a kind of emptiness that haunted him at his core. On Grieg's terms, he 'became' his mental illness: that is, whatever self he had dissipated into his obsessions and the confusion and alienation they wrought.

It is evident that, in a manner consistent with traditional, existential, psychoanalytic, rehabilitative and phenomenological literature on schizophrenia, both men felt anguish and proved dysfunctional at times. And it is no doubt likely that these men were vulnerable to psychosis in some form or another. There may have been excessive synaptic pruning, neurotoxic amino acids, loss of brain tissue, constitutional barriers to forming relationships with parents, abnormal EEG, obstetric complications, destabilizing social pressures, or even disruptions at the level of basic perceptual, worldly attunement. That said, we would still like to know what transpired such that once vital, purposive selves *found themselves* diminishing over time, until that very diminishment began to inflect whatever sense of self remained.

Here then is a principal concern in what follows. What is transpiring when people experience their own diminishment in the context of schizophrenia? How does it occur, and with what effects? If we are to address these questions, however, we first need to explore how sense of self arises in the first place.

Endnotes

1 Though developed in a different context, Peter Strawson's distinction between reactive and objectivating attitudes makes a similar point (Strawson, 1974). Whereas the latter does not acknowledge any reflexive or purposive dimension in the behavior of its subject matter, the former presumes that its subject matter is in part a meaningful site of experience and agency (and hence responsibility). One might say, then, that we are arguing that one should interpret schizophrenia from the standpoint of a reactive attitude, for it preserves what objectivating attitudes erase, namely, the view (a) that schizophrenia is a phenomenon that particular people interpret and engage in the course of their lives, and (b) that how they undergo schizophrenia in particular is a part of their particular illness.

2 Consistent with this view, Parnas and Handest (2003) find an elemental lack of attunement to the world among people with schizophrenia, which makes even basic engagement impossible. They describe, for instance, someone in the early stages of disorder, who 'tended to lose the sense of whose thoughts originated in whom and felt as if his interlocutor somehow 'invaded him', an experience that shattered his identity and was intensely anxiety provoking' (p. 129).

Chapter 3

The self in and as dialogue

So far we have reviewed two bodies of literature regarding schizophrenia. The first concerns the biological and social forces which are involved in the onset and course of the illness, while the latter, both directly and indirectly, reflects upon 'sense of self' among those living with the disease. With regard to the first set, we have argued that for all their power these courses of study tend to neglect the first-person dimensions of schizophrenia, namely, how the symptoms and challenges posed by the illness are disclosed to as well as interpreted and addressed by the person who is experiencing them. Our second review gathered numerous observations from diverse theoretical perspectives in order to sketch the experiences of diminishment that seem part and parcel of schizophrenia. We found people who regarded themselves as diminished in a variety of ways, for example, with regard to social relationships or strong emotions, and so had a sense of themselves as broken, even absorbed by their own mental illness, as in the case of Grieg.

Because we'd like to explore how one's sense of self could suffer such a fate, we first need to explore how sense of self emerges, that is, how it is that we as human beings are disclosed to ourselves outside of psychosis. To that end, we now will thicken our understanding of sense of self. With that in hand, we can turn to how such disclosures might acquire the kind of character we saw in Chapter 2.

Let's begin with a hypothesis that governs our inquiry. Human beings engage in, even live as an ensemble of dialogues. Said otherwise, the locus of life that we are, and from which the first-person emerges, is dialogical. We relate to others and ourselves, we plan, imagine, remember, and lust *only* on the basis of dialogical relations. We are thus more than an atomistic entity. In elusive but crucial ways, our being is bound to and in some sense involves the presence of others, and our lives unfold as movements within ourselves and among others.

Even at the outset, it is crucial to note that we are not claiming simply that selves employ narratives that synthesize their lives and that these narratives involve dialogues among various facets of a life. No doubt this happens to varying degrees, and we shall try to explain, at least in part, why and how, but our claim runs further than this. At base, the very self whose life one might gather up and redirect through a narrative is dialogical *in the first place*, and thus a multiple phenomenon in and of itself, not simply in its self-presentations.

What follows does not provide a comprehensive account of the self. A comprehensive theory would identify and explain elements whose interactions constitute human being, as well as the principles that govern those interactions. Such a view would have to reckon with a vast array of phenomena, from perception and self-awareness to an infant's journey into adulthood, from language and labor to emotion and conscience. It would recognize that human beings are not simply instantiations of an *eidos* or Platonist form, but unique, active loci of a temporally woven life. That said, our claim is nevertheless a strong one – dialogical relations are integral to the self, and those relations form an irreducible field out of which a sense of self is allowed to emerge.

Self as dialogue

The roots of dialogism

Because dialogical theory is far from a mainstream perspective, we will briefly sketch its roots. Among a distinguished group, we find Bakhtin's reading of Dostoyevsky, Nietzsche's reflections on subjectivity, and Dewey and Mead's social psychology particularly helpful, though we also draw heavily upon Heidegger's *Dasein*-analysis.[1] In an interpretation of Dostoyevsky's poetics, Bakhtin (1929/1985) suggests that humans are best described as polyphonic beings composed of ongoing dialogues between distinct voices. As an illustration, consider Dostoyevsky's description of Roskolnikov in *Crime and Punishment*: 'sullen, gloomy, arrogant, proud … insecure … magnanimous and kind … cold and callous … always in a hurry, always too busy and yet he lies there doing nothing' (Dostoyevsky, 1866/1993, p. 215). Bakhtin's point is not that these are contradictory modes of a singular character, but that Roskolnikov's character is an evolving movement among complementary, contrary, and even contradictory facets.

An admirer of Dostoyevsky's psychological insights, Nietzsche also describes the self as a 'subjective multiplicity'. He argues that the self is best described as a 'common wealth' or 'a social structure composed of many souls' (1886/1966, p. 26), offering the analogy that one person no more contains a singular self than Great Britain is a singular person. While the self and Britain may define themselves by certain events (e.g. a job or a long-standing commitment to liberalism), both are composed of disparate elements that cannot be synthesized without remainder. At base, the claim is phenomenological. When observing one's feelings, thoughts, and behavior, one does not find a singular entity, but an ensemble that often seems disconnected, even contentious, e.g., self-as-outgoing and self-as-introverted, or self-as-business-executive and self-as-gun-collector.

The psychology of the self-positions

In its origins, then, dialogical theory offers a self that is a complex ensemble of interanimating parts whose interactions are not driven by an overarching ego. Recently, Nietzsche and Bakhtin's view has been taken up and subjected to more systematic inquiry, and this notion of a multiplicity of souls has been cast in terms of multiple self-positions, e.g., self-as-brother or self-as-anxious. Hermans alone (1996a, 1996b) and with colleagues (Hermans, Rijks and Kempen, 1993) has studied internal dialogue as manifest in structured interviews. He concluded that one gains a sense of self when individually identifiable aspects or voices, termed 'self-positions', converse with one another, and without ever collapsing into one, overarching position. Analyzing individual patterns of verbalized self-presentation, Hermans suggests that dialogue occurs in temporary hierarchical arrangements of self-positions that periodically and spontaneously realign themselves, with dominant self-positions retreating into the background and previously subordinate self-positions coming forward. For example, suppose one is teaching a night class in a continuing education program, and one's therapist enrolls. In the classroom, self-as-teacher will have to come to the fore whereas self-as-client will have to recede, and visa-versa during sessions. Or, in order not to be a pedantic nuisance, a professor might need to move from self-as-educator to self-as-neighbor or self-as-gardener in order to establish friendships with others who live in the surrounding houses or apartments. Regardless, the point is that sense of self arises in orderly shifts and movements among multiple positions, rather than in discrete perceptions of a core state or substance.

We are drawn to the language of self-position because it offers a grammar for sense of self. On this view, sense of self involves a disclosure that presents the self-as-X. From the first-person, then, I encounter myself as subject to various determinations, e.g., self-as-hungry, self-as-consumer, or self-as-good. Not that these encounters involve intellectual intuition, i.e., an unmediated grasp of the state of our being. Recall that 'sense of self' names the manner in which we find ourselves. And as several thinkers since Kant have argued, we find ourselves always already ensconced and immersed in determinate, worldly situations. Put negatively, one never simply finds oneself determined in a single, isolated manner, as if one self-position exhausted one's being. Rather, one always finds oneself in a particular environment at a particular time involved in particular activities, and so forth. For example, one may find oneself a brother, but that encounter will always occur in a particular place, at a particular time of one's life, and in the context of particular actions, e.g., on vacation, visiting a parent, etc. We insist, therefore, that self-positions are worldly phenomena, that is, context inflected.[2]

In tying sense of self to worldly self-positions, we are committing ourselves to the view that it is something of an ongoing process of discovery or revealing, and thus a task of sorts, which can assume many forms, including but not limited to explicit practices of self-knowledge. We thus don't share Richard Rorty's (1989) conviction that a decentered account of the self dispenses with a notion of self-discovery. We agree that humans lack a fixed, ahistorical essence, but one's historically evolving and malleable being may still be something one discovers in the course of worldly interactions rather than simply fashions, and to acknowledge this is not to suppose that self-positions are necessities. No doubt they are open to interpretation and a variety of responses. For example, one may argue with one's siblings over the meaning of that relation, and one might strive to revise family structures in order to be more inclusive. Our only point, then, is a phenomenological one. As it arises (or is disclosed) in human life, sense of self is a receptive, responsive occurrence.

Let us further explore the concept of self-position. Using semi-structured interviews, Gregg (1995) also observes that regular shifts within self-awareness provide one with a sense of self. His focus, however, concerns the 'places' that might allow such shifts to occur, labeling them 'multistable or structurally ambiguous' symbols (p. 617). For example, 'diamond in the rough' could be a multistable symbol that allows one to move among differing self-descriptions such as 'crude', 'dirty', 'precious', and 'refined.' The point is not that 'diamond in the rough' absorbs these self-descriptions. Rather, like Bakhtin, Gregg holds that the self is a matter of movement and negotiation among characteristics. He thus regards these multistable symbols as elements of a narrative that enable and sustain movement and negotiation.

Although Gregg does not use this language, we read multistable symbols as self-positions in their own right. Our reasoning begins with a phenomenological reconstruction. Across one's life, various self-positions interact with one another, thus creating opportunities for generalizations about our lives with regard to those positions. If, for example, one performs well in a variety of social roles (e.g. student, athlete, and piano player), one may come to regard oneself as a 'success'. Or, if one tends to live in the moment, moving from relation to relation, one might regard oneself as a 'rolling stone'. Over time, life histories, to the degree that we weave them, gather around many such symbols. One simultaneously may regard oneself as a success, as lonely, or as a coward, and these symbols can no doubt come into contact and conflict with one another. Self-as-success, when confronted with self-as-lonely, may shrink in scope, leaving one as self-as-success with regard to solo activities but self-as-failure with regard to social ones. Second, as time moves, multistable symbols will have to engage emergent self-positions, for example, self-as-parent. Given this possibility of dialogue among multistable symbols, and dialogue between existent multistable symbols and emergent character-positions, we think it reasonable to also regard these integrating symbols as self-positions, as aspects of the self that belong to and participate in (rather than reign over) an ensemble of positions continually on the move.

While the multistable symbols Gregg locates may be regarded as self-positions, they are self-positions of a special sort: they directly refer to other self-positions. Unlike self-positions, such as self-as-brother or self-as-student, self-as-success arises through an explicit synthesis of other self-positions. True, self-as-brother implicates other positions, e.g., self-as-son, but playing that role need not require one to explicitly take up being a son. Self-as-success, however, is explicitly concerned with those positions wherein one has met with success.

Two kinds of self-positions

Given the presence of multistable symbols which nevertheless can function as self-positions in their own right, it seems justifiable to distinguish at least two kinds of self-position: 'character-positions' and 'meta-positions'. On the one hand, character-positions are self-positions like self-as-citizen, self-as-daughter, and self-as-female that stand as roles that we find ourselves inhabiting. They can be regarded as characters we play in the dramas of our lives, though we need not, and usually do not, experience them as such. Instead, they are just facets of our being.[3] Other positions, however, involve assessments of our performance within some set of roles, and these we term 'meta-positions', albeit only in a grammatical sense. The point is not that meta-positions reflect the insight or activity of a self that floats above the many self-positions whose negotiation we are. Rather, such self-positions are 'meta-positions', because they are about other self-positions, that is, they reflect one's feel for one's fate.

Of course, not everything that one undergoes becomes a self-position. Riding a bus usually will not reflect the presence of a self-position, self-as-bus-rider – but it might, since self-positions are defined functionally. A character-position involves a recurring action-orientation characteristic of one's being in the world, e.g., citizen and lover. If one often commuted by bus, and acquired the habits that orient the riding of busses, it might make sense, in order to specify how one was a 'commuter' (itself a possible character-position), to speak of self-as-bus-rider. Just riding a bus, however, would not indicate the presence of such a character-position. As far as meta-positions are concerned, they arise in reflective apprehensions of the conduct of life. If some symbol is to become a meta-position, therefore, it must be given as such in a moment of reflection, i.e., one must undergo the explicit discovery that one's being has this character. After ten years or so of commuting by bus, we could imagine, therefore, that the activity might come to stand for a kind of life, much like 'worker' connotes a kind of class-consciousness, or 'artist' names a vocation. It is thus possible that self-as-bus-rider might function as a multistable symbol capable of synthesizing a period or the whole of one's life, and so become a meta-position.

We would like to stress the irreducibly first-person dimensions of self-positions. 'Self-as-X' involves the disclosure of some state of affairs, e.g., self-as-parent, self-as-gay, to a being whose life is unfolding in those very affairs. Accordingly, self-positions are inherently reflexive phenomena, and thus categorically unlike the qualities of objects, say the green top of a table. (This presumes, of course, that 'being green' does not appear to the table as the disclosure of one of its ways of being.) In looking for self-positions, then, one cannot limit oneself to a third-person perspective and expect to find them.

We do not, however, take inherent reflexivity to signal complete disclosure or even accuracy. Again, we are not given to ourselves whole cloth in intellectual intuitions. Rather, self-positions arise out of the very life that they disclose, and in at least three ways. First, they bear the stamp of the worldly context in which they arise, one full of eco-social meanings and forces, e.g., on an oxygen-poor summit that one has ascended with one's extended family as a single, middle-aged male. Second, they arise amid and inevitably reflect some of the purposive strivings of a human life, e.g., being on vacation, running an experiment, arguing with a friend, answering a personal ad, etc. Finally, self-positions unveil time-slices within a life that is still unfolding.

They thus disclose fates whose final chapter has yet to be written. A self-position is thus as much a call for further inquiry as it is a discovery. But then, 'inquiry' may be misleading given that the self-disclosive reflexivity of self-positions is integral to our being, not simply the cast of certain explicit actions like inquiry. As Heidegger (1927/1962) aptly puts it, we are and remain questions for ourselves. The course of our life is a question for us, and the discoveries we make in that direction pose further questions.

Dialogues without authors

In order to think about how we as human beings have a sense of self that could be affected in schizophrenia, we have suggested that we are disclosed to ourselves through orderly movements among self-positions. We have also claimed that self-positions should not be regarded as modes of some deeper, core self. Instead, each is like a star in a constellation – the whole, in effect, apprehended because of interanimating plays among the parts. Of course, we know that many will resist this claim. They might agree that we present ourselves to ourselves in varied ways, and thus appear as a 'multiplex', to use Flanagan's (1994) language, but that multiplex is simply the varied appearance of a unified phenomenon. This is not our position, and primarily because we cannot find any evidence of this supposedly unified phenomenon. As Hume (1734/1888) argues, we have no knowledge of ourselves as having any 'perfect identity and simplicity', as being a kind of being that exists independently of its activities (p. 251). He continues:

> I never catch *myself* at any time without a perception, and never can observe any thing but the perception … I may venture to affirm of the rest of mankind, that they are nothing but a bundle or collection of perceptions, which succeed each other with an inconceivable rapidity, and are in a perpetual flux and movement.

> (p. 252)

Of course, in this context, our concern is self-positions, not perceptions. Moreover, a self-position is an apperceptive phenomenon. It is a matter of the perception of oneself in the midst of experience, and yet, when we try to locate a substantive or singular ego beyond any and all self-positions, we find ourselves in a place somewhat similar to the one Hume found when he attempted to introspectively locate the self. True, 'sense of self' grammatically invokes the images of someone who senses, but phenomenological reflection suggests that such reference is specious with regard to any substantial entity. In fact, Emerson seems more phenomenologically perspicacious when he writes: 'Man is a stream whose source is hidden. Our being is descending into us from we know not whence' (Porte and Morris, 2001, p. 163).

In a way, our argument is akin to one of Nietzsche's objections to Descartes. Descartes rightly concludes that the existence of doubt indicates the existence of something that is in doubt, but he was overhasty to conclude that doubts or dubious thoughts are the acts of some thinking thing, which is their agential source. Do we really summon a particular thought, like an owner calls a dog? Once again, the claim is phenomenological, and in a manner freed from the kind of grammar-driven arguments that often lead one to grope about for a transcendental ego. Thoughts, feelings, and even the insights that form the basis of meta-positions, as they are given or disclosed, come to us rather than respond to our summons, and without any apparent author. As Nietzsche (1966/1886) famously observes: 'a thought comes when *it* wishes, not when *I* wish' (p. 24). Or, as Emerson would have it: 'I conceive of man as always spoken to from behind and unable to turn his head and see the speaker' (Porte and Morris, 2001, p. 87).

Galen Strawson (2004) presents 'self-experience' as 'one's experience of oneself when one is considering oneself principally as an inner mental entity or "self" of some sort' (p. 429). Obviously, this view runs counter to ours on several fronts – for example, 'inner' versus 'worldly' – but the real bone of contention lies with the claim that introspection reveals an 'entity' that is a 'self of some sort'. Perhaps 'contention' says too much. One cannot cleanly resolve a debate if the evidence that proves decisive for one view is not available to all interlocutors. Not that there is nothing to say at the point where our view conflicts with Strawson's. We can always ask one another to look again, we can underscore what in our experience compels us to adopt one view over another, and we can genealogically explore the roots of what might seem like common sense. However, such exchanges do not empower one party to simply declare the other mistaken, and so we do not note our disagreement with Strawson in order to demonstrate the error of his ways. Rather, we note it in order to ask our readers to look and see for themselves how they find themselves to be, and to observe that philosophical psychology admits stark differences that are not easily resolvable with simple appeals to experience.

A third kind of self-position

We have been elaborating the nature and scope of self-positions, which compose the dialogues that give us a sense of self. We have aimed to establish that sense of self occurs when one encounters oneself in movements among character-positions and meta-positions. Our elaboration is incomplete, however, for we haven't presented the full range of self-positions. At times, we find ourselves threatened, and in a manner that exceeds a particular character location. One may be with friends, and thus have a sense of oneself as a friend, and encounter a physical threat that extends beyond self-as-friend. Instead, one's life is threatened; not just oneself as friend, but also one's being in general.

Phenomena like feeling threatened compel us to posit a third kind of self-position, what we will term organism-positions.[4] In these instances, the self encounters itself as it performs basic elemental functions, for example, monitoring energy levels or the relative safety of one's environment. Imagine a situation in which a fight or flight reaction occurs. In this instance, at a pre-reflective level, one senses oneself as threatened and responds with a strong disposition to either flee or confront the threat. Once again, one can interpret and respond to this encounter, but this is nevertheless an event in which one's being is disclosed to itself. It is part of the conversation. Neuroscience suggests that in flight–fight scenarios the brain functions quite differently. Higher cortical functions involving the prefrontal cortex become less involved, yet there is still a self being experienced. People can be aware during those experiences and certainly deal with them afterwards.

We take 'organism-positions' to name the kind of phenomena that Antonio Damasio (1999) associates with 'core consciousness', namely, the pre-reflective monitoring of an organism's being-in-the-world in any given here and now. We are sympathetic with Damasio's account because he regards core consciousness as thoroughly worldly – that is, it arises when an organism interprets the impact of its environment upon itself – and yet, we resist the term or metaphor of 'core' consciousness because organism-positions can and often do come into dialogue with other positions. Consider the following example. A group of male friends loiter outside a bar. Suddenly, they are aggressively accosted by another group of men. Startled and threatened, many feel a strong inclination to flee. In this instance, we would find the emergence of the organism position, 'self-as-threatened'. Now, it turns out that those who feel strongly inclined to flee also feel the tug of loyalty to their friends, that is, they are caught between self-as-threatened and the character-position, self-as-friend. Not that they deliberate, though one might. Rather, seeing the faces of their friends in similar straits leads them to remain. While dramatic, this example illustrates how organism-positions can enter into interanimating play with character-positions, and perhaps even be trumped by them when push comes to shove. We thus don't regard organism-positions as forming a core around which other positions accrue. Rather, they are one star in an interanimating constellation, which includes worldly scenarios.

We hope that we have clearly outlined the character of self-positions. On our view, they name phenomena that concretely render the grammar of our sense of self. Self-as-character-position (e.g. brother), self-as-meta-position (e.g. mediocre), and self-as-organism-position (e.g. threatened) mark out three ways in which we are given to ourselves, as Table 3.1 shows.

Let us reiterate, however, that even though we term them self-positions, each is enmeshed in worldly scenarios. Self-positions and the sense of self they afford us are thus neither purely subjective nor purely objective, but phenomena that arise when selves and their world interact. When we are disclosed to ourselves, such events do not occur in a private theater of the mind, therefore, but in the midst of our being in the world.

Table 3.1 Three forms of self-position

Type of self-position	Organism-position	Character-position	Meta-position
Description	Pre-reflective disclosures concerning the welfare of the organism	Pre-reflective disclosures concerning action-orientations derived from social roles.	Reflective disclosures concerning the overall character of parts or the whole of one's life.
Examples	Self-as-threatened, self-as-hungry, self-as-enraged, etc.	Self-as-brother, self-as-citizen, self-as-heterosexual, etc.	Self-as-success, self-as-victimized, self-as-fortunate, etc.

Self-positions in dialogue

How precisely do self-positions work in the lives they help structure and carry out? How does sense of self come to pass from one moment to the next? Let's consider that question before saying more about how sense of self emerges out of their interaction or interanimating play. Although we regard self-positions as involving an irreducibly first-person dimension, they usually are not reflective achievements. Predictably, then, we also do not take self-positions to be instances of what some call propositional attitudes.[5] Character and organism-positions have propositional content that can be evaluated, but they do not take place as judgments. We cannot make this point strongly enough. Yes, self-as-friend presumes the existence of another who somehow satisfies the conditions for being a friend, but 'being a friend' and finding oneself 'befriended' do not occur as discursive judgments about oneself and another. Instead, they occur in a wide range of actions, some of which may be self-reflective judgments. Moreover, that mesh of actions establishes the scene that one then evaluates, should the need or interest arise.

In a way, our reasoning is in line with that of Heidegger (1929/1993). Judgments are rendered upon states of affairs only after they have already been disclosed. In other words, the assertoric content of a judgment (i.e. those things and events in the world to which it refers) does not exclusively originate with the judgment, but is precisely that to which the judgment responds. One can see this in organism-positions. One finds oneself threatened, and, should there be time, one might reflect on whether the threat is genuine, but finding oneself in such a position precedes the explicit judgment. Similarly, character-positions follow suit. I don't judge myself to be a sibling and then set about being one.

What about meta-positions? They seem to explicitly have the form of a judgment, such as self-as-failure, but note that even reflective phenomena do not fall under the control of an observing, willing self. Like most of our reflective stances on things, meta-positions dawn on us, perhaps even claim us, like when we say: 'I can't escape the feeling that I'm just going about this all wrong.' Or: 'There I was, teaching, and I suddenly realized, I was a fraud.' Second, the affirmative dimension of a disclosure in which we feel like a failure is structurally different from whatever affect accompanies the judgment, 'X is a failure'. Again, not that the former lacks propositional content. Rather, the point is that when one feels like a failure, the feeling is the mode of disclosure, as opposed to the discovery of a predicate that seems to apply to a subject.

Self-positions as habits

We might put our view in yet another way. Self-positions are not merely a matter of how we perceive ourselves, but of what and how we are. How then *are* we? While we agree with Hume that we lack any singular essence or substantive ego hovering about our self-positions, in place of his bundle of perceptions, we would rather speak of a bundle of habits, agreeing with Dewey (1922/1988) that: 'All habits are demands for certain kinds of activity; and they constitute the self' (p. 21).

We are drawn to a language of habits for several reasons. First, the language of habit captures the pre-reflective nature of most human activity, from walking to shaking hands. Even movement among self-positions seems to occur without self-conscious choice. When walking down the street in a foreign city, for example, one inhabits the role of tourist, most likely behaving in ways that do not call attention to myself. If one suddenly and unexpectedly sees a friend, however, one may begin to wave and smile and act as a 'friend', and all without having 'decided' to leave self-as-tourist behind in favor of self-as-friend. The point, then, is that, for the most part, we live on autopilot. As Nietzsche (1887/1974) writes: 'For we could think, feel, will, and remember, and we could also "act" in every sense of the word, and yet none of all this would have to "enter our consciousness" (as one says metaphorically)' (p. 297). Now, one may find Nietzsche's remark exaggerated. If we take his language of consciousness to name self-consciousness, we do not.[6] Athletic and musical performances involve extremely complex behaviors, but as many have testified, heightened self-awareness during these moments or the self-conscious election of movements or actions while performing, even in virtuoso performance, is not only not required, but often is a hindrance. It would appear, then, that inhabiting and moving among self-positions occurs pre-reflectively, and drives the self in a habitual manner.

The language of habits also merges self-positions with desire and activity and clarifies how self-positions function in human behavior. Consider, for example, the habit of gambling. 'Self-as-gambler' marks a set of capacities (I know how to gamble), a set of desires (I seek the ends associated with gambling, even if not wholeheartedly), and an objective tendency to engage in those activities. Or, consider the self in an affective and meta-positional manner. 'Self-as-angry' marks a set of capacities (e.g. to yell, seek revenge, interfere, etc.), desires (e.g. to frighten, to harm, to undermine, to release steam), and an objective tendency to get angry. On our view, then, self-positions are bound to motivation and action, more as a matter of the pragmatics of subjectivity than propositional content concerning oneself, and it is principally because self-positions are bound to what Dewey terms an 'inherent tendency to action' that we regard them as habits.

It is perhaps worth stressing that not only character-positions operate habitually. Meta-positions are habitual as well. While the position 'self-as-success' may emerge in a reflective moment, it needn't remain merely reflective. In the spirit of James's (1897/1956) *The Will to Believe*, and as much self-esteem research suggests, positive self-regard may lead one to try new and novel things, that is, it is tied to a disposition to act in certain ways. For example, the meta-position 'self-as-success' could involve a range of activities in which one has been and expects to be successful.

It is important to note that we are not claiming that each action flows from a single self-position and the habits associated with it. No doubt most action is the result of multiple self-positions. Thus, for example, self-as-courageous may combine with self-as-success and, with regard to self-as-softball player, produce a risk-taking approach to softball; whereas self-as-success might combine with self-as-socially insecure and, with regard to self-as-ballroom dancer, produce a risk-aversive approach.

One might also regard organism-positions as habitual. In so far as the responses they entail reflect pre-reflectively operative dispositions to action, they function like habits as conceived by Dewey. For example, if one finds oneself chilled every fall as the temperature begins to drop, one's being pre-reflectively arrives with dispositions to act, for example, to grab a sweater. Not that organism-positions are somehow physiological habits, whereas character-positions are cultural habits. That one feels chilled every fall may have as much to do with style of dress as with falling temperatures, or one's having gotten used to hot days and warm nights. Fifty degrees Fahrenheit feels balmy in January but quite chilly in late August.

Our final reason for regarding self-positions as habits involves the way in which the concept 'habit' draws self-positions outside some well-demarcated inner realm. Bound to rhetoric of representation, self-interpretation, and even self-perception, there is a danger of seeing self-positions simply as ideas that we have about ourselves. Once self-positions are construed along the lines of habits, however, the capacities they involve are bound to the worldly scenarios that solicit and sustain them. The self-position 'self-as-gambler' will not arise unless there are situations in which one can gamble. Likewise, the self-position 'self-as-melancholic' will not arise unless loss, death, and the passage of time are in some sense there for one to dwell upon. We thus agree with Dewey that habits and, thereby, self-positions:

> may be profitably compared to physiological functions like breathing, digesting. The latter are, to be sure, involuntary, while habits are acquired. But … habits are like functions … in requiring the cooperation of organism and environment.

(1988, p. 15)

Now, one should not construe a habit's cooperation with its environment in epistemically secure terms, as if grounding in a habit insured that self-positions were the result of reliable, pre-reflective knowledge of the world. Rather than championing a kind of animal faith at the root of self-positions, our point is that habits are dependent on worldly relations. They are interactional, the feature of a being whose life is structurally bound to and reflective of engagements with a surrounding world. Thinking of self-positions in terms of habits brings them out into the world such that any given self-position is a function of and a contributing force to a thoroughly relational phenomenon.

If one takes self-positions to operate in a more or less habitual manner, it becomes evident that our being in the world is initially and primarily a matter of doing. This has implications for sense of self. If self-positions constitute the field upon which sense of self emerges, then that sense of self does not initially or usually arise in a series of observation statements about our being taken as an object. Rather, the self is disclosed to itself with regard to how it fares in its activities. As Gadamer (1981) would have it, quoting Aristotle, *praxis* names the basic way in which our *bios*, our way of life, manifests itself.[7]

The social nature of habits and dialogue

Self-positions, whose interanimating play enables sense of self, are not simply intrapersonal events. They are interpersonal as well. Said otherwise, one's internal polyphony develops and moves in response to social demands. As Emerson (1964/1836) says: 'What do we not owe to the call which society makes upon the slumbering abilities of each individual?' (p. 18). First, character-positions are bound to social roles like 'student', 'sibling', and 'parking lot attendant.'[8] We speak of 'social roles', because individuals do not create but inherit these positions. They are thus 'social' as opposed to individual. Moreover, the community at large distinguishes them from other positions in ways that are normatively binding in a loose sense. Positions like 'student' are thus not only socially generated, but what is generated amounts to a cluster of practices, expected behaviors and outcomes, the performance of which involves discernable social actions, for example, enrolling and possibly attending classes, satisfying requirements, and graduating. Not that character-positions are thoroughly rule-governed. Some roles are relatively circumscribed by the practices they entail, but in each instance, one has to acquire a kind of competence with regard to what the role requires.

While constitutive of the self, social roles are nevertheless personal, or better still, *personalized*. If only for survival's sake, social roles must be individuated by those who play them. One may be a carnivore but have learned to avoid certain meats that upset one's stomach. Also, through interaction with other self-positions, social roles cannot help but be personalized. For example, an orphan with siblings is adopted into a family without children that later becomes wealthy. These changing circumstances will individuate the manner in which she is a 'daughter'. She begins as daughter/sibling-as-orphan, then daughter/sibling-as-orphan-adopted only child, then daughter/sibling-as-orphan-adopted only child and heir to a fortune. While character-positions are bound to social roles, their relation is a true relation and not a unidirectional process of construction.

The sociality of self-positions is evident in another manner: their place in one's self-organization is often influenced by the regard or recognition of others. As Hegel (1807/1979) noted, and as others have more recently argued (Mackenzie, 2000; Oliver, 2002), our self-conscious self-regard is vulnerable to the contradictory regard of others. Moreover, we often need the acknowledgement or recognition of others in order to imagine ourselves becoming the person we take ourselves to be, or who we would like to be. (In a way, the regard of others is really just one facet of the worldly situation in which self-positions arise.)

If you ask a question at a lecture, or if you present a request to a clerk, should everyone look at you as if you were speaking gibberish, it will be difficult to persist in that line of inquiry. Similarly, if you are continually given the impression that you are unfit to assume certain tasks, it will be quite difficult to believe that you can, whereas the confidence of others can a go a long way towards giving us confidence in ourselves.

The presence or absence of recognition has obvious implications for meta-positions. One may take oneself to be a success, but if one's communication of that belief meets with incredulity or even scorn, it will prove increasingly difficult to maintain the meta-position. Similarly, if the range of one's character-positions is continually denigrated, maintaining positive self-regard will prove onerous. Recognition is also relevant to character-positions in and of themselves. As we've suggested, one grows into character-positions though habituation. One is unlikely to begin that process, however, or fare well in it, if one is given the strong impression, either explicitly or implicitly, that one has no business becoming a doctor or professor, for example. Interestingly, recognition may even be relevant with regard to organism-positions. As noted, the confidence that another has in us may buoy our own belief in our capabilities. If so, a situation might initiate an organism-position, e.g., self-as-anxious, that subsides with the explicit or implicit reassurance of another, say through a focused look and smile, or a pat on the back.

The dialogical origins of life histories

Thus far our focus has been the pre-reflective operations of self-positions, but sense of self is also related to reflectively generated life histories. How though does a dialogical self come to reflectively regard itself and generate life histories as well as the meta-positions that anchor them? In order to answer this question, we will make use of Jürgen Habermas's (1981, 1988) reading of George Herbert Mead.

Habermas's work focuses in part on the logic and sociality of communication or what he terms 'communicative action' (i.e. action oriented towards mutual understanding). A source of social integration, communication enables us to coordinate actions. If it is to do so, however, one needs to know what another is going to do, and as an individual, not as a generic 'brother', 'professor', or 'customer'. Learning to communicate involves, therefore, learning to meet an expectation performatively intrinsic to communication, to speak for oneself as a singular being. One finds a similar expectation when we are called to communicate our needs. The expression of needs requires speech acts in the first-person. If I am to receive what I want or you are to provide me with what I need, I must make my needs plain to you. These no doubt will be bound to social roles, that is, many of my needs will arise vis-à-vis character-positions, but unless I can express myself in the first-person, they will only be met ineffectively.

Not only expressive speech acts require the first-person, however. In fact, all speech acts do. Even when one refers to impersonal events, such as how many miles lie between Eugene, Oregon and Ghent, Belgium, one is still expected to provide reasons for one's beliefs should others find them puzzling, and the same holds for conduct. In communicative action, we are expected to answer for what we say, do, and believe, and strictly speaking, others cannot answer for us. Should someone answer for us, we will still be asked, 'is that what you meant?'

We have dipped into Habermas's theory of communicative action because it shows how, in acquiring communicative competencies, we not only acquire linguistic capacities but modes of self and other relation that encourage and even require us to adopt a first-person perspective. Integrating his view with ours, the claim is that the 'I' of first-person speech becomes a structural element in all self-positions, one dialogically tethered to actual and possible interlocutors and grounded in the habits required for communicative competence. In other words, the 'I' of first-person speech, that which we identify with ourselves, is a dialogical phenomenon. It is neither a source of agency nor spontaneous judgment – those are tied to the habits that collect around and constitute other self-positions. It is an acquired capacity for self-regard that amounts to an internalized sense of another's regard for one, a regard that less interjects some content-rich identity than expects one to answer for what one says and does.

On Habermas's view, and here we follow him, our communicative capacity for self-regard lies at the root of life histories. Meta-positions arise when we tell the story of our lives to others and/or ourselves. Looking forwards and backwards, we capture our fate and expectations with a range of multistable symbols that reflectively synthesize lives we have lived and some we would like to live. This capacity has an interpersonal root, however. Communicative competence entails learning how to answer for one's beliefs and actions. It thus demands a self-interrogation whose fruits can be shared with and scrutinized by others, say by being expressed linguistically. Communicative competence is thus an enabling condition for the kind of reflective dialogical activity that a life history requires, and for the generation of meta-positions in particular.

Interestingly, integrating Habermas's theory of communicative action with a dialogical theory of the self allows us to see how life histories are thoroughly dialogical and not the product of a central, authorial ego. First, their subject matter concerns the various self-positions within which our life unfolds. As a narrative, a life history thus involves a dialogue among these positions. Second, life histories are not generated by some amorphous 'I'. Rather, and this repeats an earlier point, to say 'I' in the context of a life history is simply to take responsibility for previous and prospective actions and beliefs. Habermas (1988) writes: 'Standing within an intersubjectively shared lifeworld horizon, the individual projects himself as someone who *vouches* for the more or less clearly established continuity of a more or less self-consciously appropriated life history' (p. 168).[9] As far as the actual telling is concerned, one will have to look again at determinate self-positions and the social locations they involve. For example, one might gather the events of one's life in therapy, or while applying for a job, or as one ages and faces a crisis of meaning. Finally, the positions from which life histories are gathered can themselves enter into dialogue with other self-positions. Thus self-as-memoirist may come into contact with self-as-truthful, or self-in-therapy may come into contact with self-as-self-sufficient. Or a life history may become a creative exercise and produce its own meta-positions, e.g., self-as-victim, which functions proactively alongside other self-positions. Life histories and the coherence they bring about are thus dialogical at the level of their formal preconditions and at the level of content. Not only do they involve a synthesis of positions, but also, one pursues them from dialogically situated positions and on the basis of a dialogically generated capacity.

Sense of self emerging

At the end of Chapter 2, we asked: how does someone come to sense that he or she is diminishing? In order to address that question, we have sought to outline how sense of self unfolds, irrespective of whether it is diminishing or flourishing. Our suggestion is that sense of self emerges through intra-and interpersonal dialogue. As a complex entity, a 'multiplicity of souls', to use Nietzsche's language, the self is disclosed to itself within interanimating plays among three kinds of self-positions: character-positions (e.g. self-as-author), organism-positions (e.g. self-as-exhausted), and meta-positions that refer to and comment upon the other kinds of self-positions, (e.g. self-as-diamond-in-the-rough). Though analytically distinct, each can engage and influence the other, and character and organism-positions can function in meta-positional ways (e.g. self-as-criminal).

Within a self, all of these self-positions bring life and meaning to one another when they interact. In their interaction, they inflect one another, as if they were stars in a constellation, the mass of each influencing how the light of each travels through the cosmos. Principally, movement among self-positions is a worldly affair, which is to say, it occurs in response to determinate circumstances and as primarily a matter of habit. Self-positions are not just ideas or principally representational phenomena. They are intertwined and partly constitute the existential praxis that informs our being-in-the-world. Their movement – which includes the human actions they help fund – does not derive from the decision of any singular self. That said, self-positions can be reflectively considered in life histories where relations between character and organism-positions are often examined and sometimes synthesized, often through the generation of multistable meta-positions. Such histories are dialogical, however, whether in the capacities that enable them, the subject matter that concerns them, or the self-positions from which they are generated.

So how does sense of self actually arise? At base, sense of self involves a disclosure of the self-as-X. The 'X' could be a character-position (self-as-brother), an organism-position (self-as-elated), or a meta-position (self-as-scheming). Such a disclosure is never an isolated occurrence. Each self-position comes to the fore in a moving and interanimating field of porous positions, each enmeshed in worldly contexts. These contexts prompt the appearance of the self-position and the sense of self that it affords, such that 'sense of self' is given as we make our way through and respond to the world. The self-positions which take place in the dialogues that define us are also organized within hierarchies which periodically shift or change. To rework some of Thomas Nagel's justly famous phrases, what it's like to be a self is never given in or to a view from nowhere (Nagel, 1974, 1986). We find ourselves always already in character and organism-positions, often in compound ways, and even when generating a meta-position. Alongside the 'sense of self' given through the meta-position one also gains a 'sense of self' through the character-position from which the meta-position in part emerges, which neatly shows how 'sense of self' can be a polyphonic occurrence.

Before turning to how this process could register diminishment and whether that mirrors what we have observed in schizophrenia, we will provide an extended illustration of how sense of self emerges from moment to moment. Imagine traveling somewhere on a plane, say to a professional meeting. You check over your things, bid your partner goodbye, and walk to the street where a cab awaits. As you get in, you wave to a neighbor, and look anxiously across the street at a group of shady characters assembling in your local park. Settling into the cab, you dramatically rehearse the scene of your presentation and feel certain that it will strike your audience as impressive.

In this brief scenario, several character-positions come into play: self-as-partner, self-as-professional, self-as-neighbor, self-as-customer, and, depending upon how one responds to the scene in the park, possibly self-as-citizen. Our claim is that each reflects a pre-reflectively operative, determinate way of being-in-the-world. Second, each arises as a response to a worldly scenario, e.g., a conference convening at some distance, being partnered, seeing a neighbor, etc. Third, each gives one a sense of oneself as being that kind of character, and in the course of conducting one's life. One might feel loved as partner, lucky as a neighbor, confident as a professional, and frustrated as a citizen, and one could imagine how this last disclosure leads you to kvetch with the taxi driver about the city's inability to deal with its persistent drug trade, as well as to an experience of gratitude for your reliable, attentive neighbors.

Let's continue our tale of traveling by plane. After a relatively effortless beginning, imagine that your trip takes a turn for the worse: plane delays, missed connections, and a late arrival. Along the way, self-as-customer and self-as-traveler come into play in relation to airline employees, one's fellow passengers, and the masses milling about the two airports you see all too much of. In these instances, character-positions again lead the way. At some point, however, you lose your temper to the point that an organism-position like self-as-frustrated appears.

Its appearance, however, is still bound to the ensemble of character-positions operative at the moment, and to the scenarios that pushed one over the edge. That is, the organism-position remains dialogically situated and worldly, a fact further evidenced by the repercussions your tantrum has for the performances still required by the persisting character-positions. Say you initially turn to fellow travelers for support, but later apologize to the gate attendant, given that she has little control over bad weather. You might even say, 'I just lost it', which we take to mean, an organism-position rushed to the fore of one's dialogical ensemble, and trumped whatever habits usually govern the performance of roles like customer and fellow traveler.

Finally, you arrive at your hotel, check in, and unwind, a process that involves recurring character-positions like self-as-customer and self-as-traveler, as well as an organism-position, self-as-tired. Looking back on the day, discussing it with your partner on the phone, a recurring meta-position arises, replete with a degree of shame, namely, self-as-impatient. After hanging up, you look ahead to the next day, and take solace in having your presentation good and ready. In fact, this recalls another meta-position, self-as-professional-success, and so you wonder how you can be so cool in certain circumstances, and such a hothead in another – but not for long, given how tired you are. In this reflective moment, several positions are in play: the character-positions in which one keeps one's cool and fails to, the character-position operative in staying in a hotel, most likely, self-as-traveler, though maybe also self-as-professional if one travels a good deal, two meta-positions, and an insistent organism-position.

Quite an ensemble, but that is the kind of complexity that underwrites our being-in-the-world, and out of which sense of self arises and evolves. Yet, for all the polyphonic richness and subsequent chance for disequilibrium that our dialogical natures entail, most people seem to pursue lives of relative stability, and to experience themselves as effective agents. On the whole, many might present themselves as subject to unresponsive institutional arrangements, and many might feel trapped in various character-positions, but few actually experience themselves as 'broken' or 'empty' or dispersed into fragments. Yet that is precisely the kind of experiences of diminishment that many undergo who suffer from schizophrenia. As Grieg remarked: 'That's the hell of it … some days you just aren't there.' Let us turn then to consider how one might come to experience oneself in this way.

Endnotes

1 In a way, there are actually two dialogical traditions. One is oriented around Buber and stresses the primary intersubjectivity of human self-experience. Another looks back to Bakhtin and focuses upon intrapsychic life as dialogical. If only at a thematic level, our view synthesizes these two perspectives, also drawing upon Nietzsche's anticipations of Bakhtin, existential phenomenology, and pragmatist social psychology.

2 Our claim presumes the relative soundness of Heidegger and Dewey's claim that humans do not exist *in* the world in the manner of a generic corporeal entity, e.g., water lying in a glass (Heidegger, 1927/1962; Dewey, 1988). Rather than simply lying beside or within the world, humans actively interpret it, and experience themselves as thoroughly involved in that world, e.g., breathing air, walking along a street, seeking a meal, admiring a sunset, etc.

3 In invoking social roles, our work builds upon views developed by Alasdair MacIntyre (1984) and Mark Johnson (1993). It no doubt also overlaps with Goffman's work on character as performance (1959).

4 In adding organism-positions to our account, and in employing the language of character-positions, we are revising the position we presented in the essay 'Being interrupted: The self and schizophrenia' (Lysaker and Lysaker, 2005).

5 The language of 'propositional attitudes' is so widespread in Anglo-American philosophy of mind that a few citations of particular articles would fail to convey the prevalence of the view that we are resisting. A better indication of the concept's place in a major strand of contemporary philosophical discourse can be found in *The Stanford Encyclopedia of Philosophy*. (The SEP is available online at http://plato.stanford.edu/.) One not only finds the term in entries on belief, emotion, and mental representation, but also in 424 other entries.

6 Damasio distinguishes between core and extended consciousness, and on his terms, the former is no doubt operative in the scenarios Nietzsche imagines. Nietzsche's concern is really reflective self-consciousness, however, so Damasio's distinction doesn't touch the heart of his observation.

7 Interestingly, we think Damasio (1999) would agree. Attention, one of the necessary conditions for core consciousness is spontaneously purposive on his view. It is thus always oriented towards some end and thus a kind of activity or praxis.

8 How one comes to inhabit roles is a complex subject for developmental psychology, and beyond our scope. No doubt many processes are operative, e.g., parental instruction, mimicry, play, internalization of expectations, etc.

9 Galen Strawson (2004) believes that some people do not and need not project themselves in terms of a life narrative. Yes, they may recall the recent past and plan for the
immediate future, but overall, their life is 'episodic' and of the moment. At one level
we agree. Not everyone novelistically recounts their lives, nor should they, but
regarding and presenting one's self as 'episodic' seems to employ a meta-position
that establishes continuity throughout a life and vouches for it. It seems then
that Strawson's effort to legitimate lifestyles that do without narrative life histories
actually employs one.

Chapter 4

Dialogical impairment and self-diminishment

In Chapter 1 we argued that exclusively third-person accounts of schizophrenia face two significant problems. If we only explore schizophrenia in terms of a volatile array of symptomatology, social barriers to wellness, and possible courses of illness, we cast those with schizophrenia as passive beings locked in flawed bodies or unjust social networks. Moreover, we rush past a first-person fact of the matter – those who suffer from schizophrenia undergo it, and how they undergo it is part of the illness. In the second chapter, we considered several writers from very different theoretical perspectives who have tried to articulate the phenomenon of schizophrenia with the first-person in play. On these accounts, to the degree they cohere, schizophrenia involves a profound disruption in self-experience. By moving beyond purely third-person accounts of schizophrenia, we found a subjectivity whose core sense of self is paradoxically centered in feelings of diminishment relative to a personal past, that is, such people feel as if they once were but no longer are effective agents in their own becoming. The quantitative metaphorics are thus quite precise.

Chapter 2 closed with questions about how one might sense one's own diminishment. In order to answer this question, it was necessary to account for how sense of self arises in the first place. We thus devoted Chapter 3 to a view of how selves are experienced when psychosis isn't present. If we can locate the sites and events whereby selves are disclosed to themselves, we should be able to investigate how one might find oneself profoundly diminished with regard to one's presence and influence in the course of one's life.

In the third chapter, we argued that sense of self does not involve the apprehension of a substantial, singular, and authorial self that resides within. The view that we have a singular, substantial self has fallen prey to a trick of grammar, or ventured a mistaken inference from a pragmatic, discursive act that facilitates communication: that is, employing the first-person pronoun. Instead, we sense ourselves within and through encounters that are at once intra- and interpersonal, and that reflect complementary and dissonant facets of our being. More precisely, sense of self emerges out of an interaction among self-positions, namely, character-positions, organism-positions, and meta-positions. Properly speaking, 'positions' are not ideas or representations of our selves. Rather, self-positions are axes of self–world interaction, more a matter of who we are, than of whom we take ourselves to be (in fact, only meta-positions emerge in reflective acts). Moreover, self-positions function more or less habitually, and this includes meta-positions once they've been formulated and have settled. Our overall claim, then, is that sense of self is dialogical, the disclosure of a being to itself through an interanimating play of multiple, often partially discontinuous self-facets within shifting worldly contexts.

In this chapter, we return to experiences of diminishment in schizophrenia and explore whether they can be accounted for by a disruption in the dialogical processes that enable sense of self in the first place. Specifically, we will suggest that if the interanimating play of self-positions were significantly compromised, one should expect to find an experience of self-diminishment very close to what is found in schizophrenia.

To make this argument, we will consider some ways in which interplay among self-positions might be compromised. We will then ask whether such compromises might lead to experiences of self-diminishment along the lines that many theorists, from various perspectives, associate with schizophrenia. After answering in the affirmative, we will concretize our account with clinical examples. Finally, we offer a general model for interpreting disturbed self-experience in schizophrenia. Throughout, we will address the fact that the experience of self-diminishment associated with schizophrenia is not an experience of lessened capacities, e.g., memory loss or weakened abstract problem-solving, but an awareness of one's own diminishment over time. Moreover, unlike in dementia, where confusion and memory loss may occur without any awareness of lessened capacities, in schizophrenia, people appear fully cognizant of their diminishment.

Dialogism and disrupted self-experience in schizophrenia

Dialogical disarray and riddled self-experience

The interanimating play that sustains sense of self occurs at multiple levels. Basic character-positions, organism-positions and meta-positions respond to one another, immediate experience, historical experience, others, recollections of others, the imagined behavior of others, and so forth. This interplay is, by definition, dynamic but nevertheless ordered, and meaning emerges from these dialogues because shifts in positions prove both responsive to worldly situations and more or less internally coherent, if occasionally dissonant. As discussed briefly in Chapter 3, Hermans (1996a; b) has hypothesized that self-positions enter into dialogue within a hierarchy that periodically shifts. For example, while talking with a group of friends after work, one may find oneself giving and kind, though also a trickster from time to time. As more non-friend colleagues join the table, group dynamics naturally shift, and so does one's behavior. Suppose that jokes and pranks increase while feelings of warmth and generosity mellow. In such cases, shifts in self-positions, as well as their perpetual interplay, flow in an orderly fashion and prove responsive to the changing situation. The result is a more or less continuous, if occasionally surprising web of experiences, i.e., nothing is particularly jarring, even though one might realize along the way that a certain co-worker is always (and unjustly) the butt of one's pranks, while another proves increasingly attractive.

Now, if a certain degree of disorder interrupted the flow of the many self-positions implied above, it is likely that one's intrapersonal dialogues would be imperiled, just as sense is hard to come by in a sentence in which all the words are said at once. If one cannot inhabit any one position or set of positions in particular, no determinate sense of self will appear. Instead, it would be as if one had fallen through the cracks.

Consider a few hypothetical examples. The first involves a scenario that, despite its exaggerated density, many will recognize as overwhelming even without the challenge of psychosis. Imagine hosting a gathering that combines a few family members, two former lovers, a present lover, some old friends, some new friends who don't know the old friends, colleagues, a supervisor, and one or two rivals who verge on being enemies. The presence of each solicits a wide range of responses and meta-positions, as well as associations which themselves solicit responses. Locked into the role of host, one does okay initially. Over time, however, one finds oneself pulled in multiple, conflicting dimensions. After sharing a conversation with one's supervisor, a deservedly angry ex-lover, and an old friend who has recently returned to town after a period of estrangement, one slips out of a crowded living room in favor of a balcony, muttering 'this is too much'. The scenario, while extreme, captures a more common feeling. Sometimes, so many facets of our being are animated (which initiates their action orientations), that we're overwhelmed, and to the point that our experience becomes an incoherent flurry of white noise. In fact, it may be that we begin to encounter ourselves only as overwhelmed. We might even feel a mild panic.

Now imagine a scenario where a similar cluster of positions are animated, but in ways that no obvious situation summons. What if the self-positions of self-as-teacher, self-as-soccer-fan, self-as-kind, self-as-opposing-authoritarian-government, and self-as-still-in-love-with-Karen, all of which were previously grounded in rich intra- and interpersonal conversations, began to emerge while one deliberated about whether to go on a diet? Here, the confusion resulting from the flurry of self-positions would be intensified by the disruption that their inappropriateness affects. Under such conditions, not only would it be difficult to make a decision about the diet or books, but without any order to the positional flow, one's sense of self would be dispersed into all the positions through which we are disclosed to ourselves. It might very well seem that everything had fallen figuratively into a heap of rubble. Multiple self-positions would remain but without organized interaction, and the emergence of new positions would only join a downward spiral towards the experience of subjective disintegration.

An inverse though related process might produce similar results. Instead of a disordered play among self-positions, what if one found oneself within a rigid hierarchy resistant to any shifts or changes? In such a state, with few self-positions or even a solitary position maintaining dominance, intra- and interpersonal dialogue would be severely limited. Keeping with the above scenario, what if dealing with ill relatives, grateful colleagues, and a politically active and humorless neighbor were all organized by self-as-opposing-authoritarian-government? In this instance, what was formerly a rich array of self-positions would be tyrannically denied entry into the conversation, and one's sense of self would appear as sustained by a lone voice (e.g., 'I am opposing tyranny'). Moreover, over time, social interactions would prove increasingly difficult insofar as they require perspectives and skills not required by anti-authoritarian protests – and such struggles could only underscore the fact that one had become a less effective presence than before.

For an even more potent example of this second process, suppose that one's intra- and interpersonal dialogue became dominated by aspects of an emerging psychosis, such that all manner of circumstances were understood through the mediation of only one self-position (e.g., self-as-persecuted or self-as-all-powerful). In a monologue of persecution, former friends might be seen as foes if they questioned the monologue, and any interaction that formerly evoked positive or loving traits would be annulled by suspicions of ulterior motives, even given evidence to the contrary. Similarly, previously entertaining events that supported aspects of self that were related to casual interests, such as going to a see a movie, would be transformed into experiences of insidious assault. Over time, such lines of self–world interaction would very likely affect sense of self. Unlike the previous cases of ramped disorder, one would retain the sense-of-self afforded by the dominant position, in these cases, meta-positions like self-as-persecuted or self-as-all-powerful; but that benefit would be taxed by the undoing of other positions. As always, multiple self-positions would arise given shifting circumstances, but without an opportunity to interanimate, they would fall by the wayside, or be translated into modes of the dominant position. One expects that these relentless translations would eventually affect an experience of diminishment, if not generate an organism-position of self-at-risk.

Interrupted dialogues and previous accounts of diminished self-experience

We have suggested that a relative loss or calcification of an ordered, interanimating play among self-positions could result in a sense of one's self as diminished. How similar would this experience be to the kinds of self-disturbances that researchers, while working from traditional psychiatric, existential, psychoanalytic, rehabilitative and phenomenological perspectives, have observed among people suffering from schizophrenia? Let's begin at the beginning. A disordered and/or rigidly arranged play of self-positions would seem to effect results that closely parallel what Bleuler and Kraeplin both identified as coincident with the objective symptoms of schizophrenia. Without temporarily stable self-locations, a person might be unable to 'orient himself either inwardly or outwardly', as Bleuler (1911/1950) observed. Without an intra- and interpersonal conversation in which different self-facets contribute and relate to different aspects of others, even a simple social milieu would prove dizzying, and if one cannot inhabit a relatively stable character-position, habitual social orientations will go missing or unhelpfully conflate. Likewise, if multiple self-facets are animated, but in an unordered fashion, one's internal landscape will seem chaotic, to the point that one could experience the 'destruction of the internal connection of the psychic personality', as Kraeplin (1919/2002) contended. On our view, intra- and interpersonal dialogues connect us with ourselves and others, and as they dim, or rather, as they prove inaccessible or unnavigable, one might very well think that the basic threads of personality had been destroyed.

Turning to the views of the existentialists, without dialogue to connect oneself to others or to connect aspects of oneself to other aspects of self, a 'rent' in intra- and interpersonal relations of the sort Laing (1978) observed would likely appear. Without fluidly ordered dialogical interactions among self-positions, people could know that they exist and remember the qualities of past relationships, but their living present would lack ongoing, reciprocal exchanges which are the essence of intersubjectivity, and their own sense of self would prove radically discontinuous with their past and fractured in their present.

In a manner consistent with Boss's (1979) perspective, our claim is that if dialogue comes to a relative halt, a person will be unable to be 'free, self-reliant and enduring' (p. 235) in the face of changing life events. As described in the examples above, a person facing a disordered or calcifying play of self-positions lacks the kind of existential axes through which humans interpret and engage the world's varying and relentless demands.

Consistent with psychoanalytic observations, such as those summarized by Frosh (1983), severe compromises in our dialogical capacities might lead us to feel on the brink of psychic destruction, if not on the far side of that cataclysm. If the interplay that provides a sense of self-relation or 'interiority' bucks and sways, one's sense of self will join the upheaval. Selzer and Schwartz (1994) note that people with schizophrenia sometimes believe they have been destroyed psychologically, but this is precisely how one would feel if every mooring for sense of self began to whirl about chaotically, or if every worldly situation were shunted into a rigid and unresponsive mode of self-presentation. Without an ordered play of self-positions, our sense of self would fall into a maelstrom. Or, if trapped within a single self-position, a formerly successful history of self–world interaction, complete with sufficient intersubjective recognition of our self-presentations, would give way to increasing social alienation. Moreover if dialogue more or less ceased, once accessible self-facets might prove irretrievable, leading one to conclude, consistent with Kraeplin's findings, that one had vanished or been destroyed. Such a result is also consistent with the sense of being 'withered' that certain phenomenologists have noted (Blankenburg, 2001), and with the observation by Stanghellini (2004) that without the dialectic between the 'I' and the 'me', individuals are vulnerable to experiencing nothingness.

The struggles that we've associated with dialogical compromises also overlap with the lack of attunement and common sense that phenomenologists like Mishara (2004) have observed among those suffering from schizophrenia. Again, without the worldly orientations that self-positions provide, subtle social rules will prove elusive. If one loses the habitually operative action orientations given with character-positions, it will be difficult to engage the world in a manner responsive to the situation in question. If one does not have a good sense of whether one is presently a customer, friend, or sexual partner, interpreting the gestures, looks, and tone of another's voice will be inordinately difficult.

Of note, our view does seem somewhat at odds with Sass (2003), who suggests that schizophrenia undermines sense of self because it involves an intensity of self-interest, which overwhelms connections with others. In our view, this intensity of self-interest or self-awareness is actually an effect of breakdowns in intra- and interpersonal dialogues, although priority is difficult to establish in such matters. With the collapse of dialogical play, self-awareness is unhinged from its moorings in an interanimating play of positions, and thus haunts psychic life like a specter in search of a home. As one self-position assumes dominance and dialogue more or less freezes, an apparent magnification of self-experience results because only one self-position is effectively in play, and in a way that renders self–world interaction precarious at best. In scenarios of unbridled disorder, there is really no determinate self-position to obsess over, and so what appears to be a turn inward is simply what remains when the ability to turn in any determinate direction is severely undermined. For example, and we'll have more to say about this in Chapter 6, someone with schizophrenia may avoid the views and affects of others because the dialogical play their presence animates threatens to overwhelm whatever modest stability had been achieved. In such a case, we might see an excess of self-experience as described by Sass, but one sustained to prevent the further destruction of self that would follow a meaningful intersubjective experience.

Finally, as detailed in Chapter 2, rehabilitation specialists (Lally, 1989; Roe and Ben-Yishai, 1999) have observed how people in the midst of schizophrenia find themselves engulfed and overwhelmed by their illness. They can only experience themselves as their illness and they define themselves as 'schizophrenic', as something less than human. Returning to Bleuler's poignant description of the man who cannot 'orient himself either inwardly or outwardly', we ask: might not someone identified by others as *being* mentally ill assume that identification if a diminishing internal dialogue left him or her bereft of any other determinate sense of self? Without an internal dialogue providing sense of self and self–world orientations, people might very well only regard themselves in terms provided them by those who treat them, particularly if those terms are also adopted by others with whom they interact (e.g., a family member reminding the person to take medicine, a therapist asking about symptoms, and employers asking if he or she needs an accommodation at work). With one's 'sense of self' crumbling, some creature comfort may be had if the person with schizophrenia weds his or her sense of self to a third-person view of his or her condition.

Finding oneself diminishing: two cases

We have suggested that either a relative loss of order or the calcification of hierarchies among self-positions could produce a sense of one's self as diminished, and in a manner that is consistent with multiple accounts of the first-person dimensions of schizophrenia. We'd now like to concretize those claims with some clinical examples, and argue that a dialogical account of self-disruption can help explain how one might remain aware of such disruptions. Let's return to the cases of Frank and Grieg that we offered at the end of Chapter 2. We knew Frank before and after the onset of schizophrenia, which enabled us, in the context of psychotherapy, to speak with him over the course of several years about his experiences with mental illness. As discussed briefly in Chapter 2, Frank came to psychotherapy as a young man struggling with issues related to love, money and education. Suddenly, following an extended vacation, he became acutely psychotic. Alongside symptoms that were the target of a pharmacological intervention, Frank presented himself in terms of 'emptiness and nothingness', precisely the kind of state we've been discussing in terms of a sense of oneself as diminished. He experienced an anguish that exceeded the feeling of being perpetually persecuted. He believed and felt that the person he once was had 'exploded', leaving him as a collection of remnants that, held together by a weak form of 'gravity', lingered in the place where he had been.

From the view we've been developing, our hypothesis is that Frank's intra- and interpersonal dialogues calcified. Specifically, with onset, Frank's self–world interactions gathered almost exclusively around a single self-position, which we would label 'self-as-persecuted'. Prior to psychosis, a wide range of character and meta-positions emerged when Frank spoke about the project of his life. He recounted experiences at college, and articulated his sense of what prevented him from returning. Along the way, he presented himself as a failed student, an angry son, a music lover, in love, etc. After onset, however, each position was absorbed into self-as-persecuted, and in a complex way. On the one hand, it overlay everything like a ubiquitous meta-position, and he would present himself as such. On the other hand, it informed every action orientation, and so named the fundamental role he played in the story of his life – the persecuted one. In fact, given the degree of anxiety and anguish this feeling of being persecuted produced, 'self-as-persecuted' verged on becoming an organism-position continually producing the desire to flee.

Once psychosis set in, the previously rich conversations that characterized Frank's psychotherapeutic sessions vanished, and the complexity of his former life appeared inaccessible to him. Yes, Frank was still angry with his father and he still loved music, but these had little purchase on his sense of self or his self–world orientation. Moreover, the predominance of 'self-as-persecuted' made engaging him nearly impossible unless one addressed the fact of his persecution. He could only talk about his impending assassination and the rage he felt towards his perceived stalkers. He could remember discussing issues related to love and work, but when offered a chance to discuss his family, his love of music, or even the possibility of someday returning to college, Frank angrily responded to these offers as hostile attempts to 'change the subject'. Now, this moment, which initiated much of the theoretical work organizing our study, made evident that, for all intents and purposes, Frank could only see himself in light of his perceived persecution. He had become 'self-as-persecuted'. His therapist, uncertain of how to proceed, noticed the anger in Frank's voice, and shared his observation. Frank replied that maybe the therapist was the 'angry one'. In return, the therapist expressed frustration with the fact that they could only discuss one topic, and that the richness of their previous exchanges had disappeared. As noted before, Frank then said that if he tried to think of anything outside of the rigid confines of his persecution, he felt emptiness and nothingness, and he went on to conclude that part of him had been destroyed.

In our view, this movement from an exclusive self-position to self-as-destroyed is predictable. With only one self-position securing self–world interactions and providing any sense of self, Frank had no other access to his welfare, even though he knew that in the past, his experiences were multidimensional and varied. Thus, when pushed beyond the confines of self-as-persecuted, he could only see an abyss to one side and the life he had lived on the other, leaving him feeling as if his once rich and varied life had been destroyed. In other words, he rather suddenly found himself less than he once was.

We should stress, however, that experiences of self-diminishment do not amount to senses of global destruction. The formal structure of one's sense of self remains – i.e., one is still disclosed to oneself in some particular way – but what is disclosed is given as a diminishment relative to what one recalls about oneself. This is what one would expect given our dialogical theory, which holds that compromises in the interanimating play that sustains dialogue do not render one unable to sense oneself, but systematically unravel determinate senses of self. This is because such compromises do not erase one's memory of previous interactions among self-positions, and thus they do not erase previous sense(s) of self. However, they do keep previous sense(s) of self abstract, a matter of who one had been rather than live possibilities, which leaves one aware of who one no longer is.

With the case of Grieg, matters are similar if less sudden. As you might recall, Grieg had been unhappy in early youth, but he had sustained attachments and followed a course of meaningful activity. He experienced himself as a person whose conflicts complicated his attempts to navigate a difficult life. He dreamt of marrying and of being a carpenter. He went to his high school prom. With the onset of psychosis in early adulthood, he suddenly lost any sense of control over his life. Where he had previously directed his own activities, he came to feel that hospitals and psychotic experiences controlled his life while he looked on, unable to meaningfully intervene, let alone take charge.

After a short period of self-diminishment, however, Grieg experienced a return to what he regarded as normality. He was soon working and attached to people. He married, had children, and once again found himself to be an effective presence in the world, but things began to decline following a tragic death in his family, and it was in regard to this period that he remarked: 'I became mental illness.' Consistent with the perspectives of some individuals from the tradition of psychiatric rehabilitation (e.g., Roe, 2001), he had vanished, leaving only an illness as his defining factor.

It strikes us that, with each onset of illness, Grieg's once rich series of intra- and interpersonal dialogical exchanges dwindled, while in the intervening periods, they recovered some of their internally diverse, interanimating play. As Grieg recounts them, pre-psychosis experiences involved positions such as self-as-son-who-disappointed-the-mother, self-as-lover-of-wife, self-as-unappreciated-worker, self-as-grateful-father, self-as-beloved-brother and self-as-future-carpenter. After onset, only a few self-positions were operative, namely, self-as-persecuted and self-as-beloved, and references to these persecuting and affirming presences contained little detail beyond their belittling and denigrating addresses, although cultural icons, speaking through the television, were sometimes the sources of praise. Under the spell of these addresses, Grieg framed all personal events and affects in terms of his impending humiliation or admiration. Yet these engagements failed to provide Grieg with any sense of his own activity, or any connection to determinate others. Eventually, there was no way for him to orient himself inward or outwardly, as Bleuler would say. We say this because, when questioned about current events in his life, including how he felt, thought, or acted in regards to daily stressors, Grieg offered responses that focused upon his impending capture, and that were virtually identical to one another, although he seemed unaware that he was repeating himself.

As with Frank, our hypothesis is that Grieg's weakening social attachments and sense that he had diminished over the course of his illness reflect a contraction of intra- and interpersonal dialogue. In place of the fluid, interanimating play of self-positions that had characterized his life before the onset of schizophrenia, Grieg moved between two parallel loops of self–world interaction that alienated him from others and gave him little sense of self beyond what his symptoms provided (unless those symptoms were presented as such by folk like health care professionals). The resulting contrast thus gave Grieg the sense that whoever he had been had disappeared into his mental illness.

A taxonomy of disturbed self-experience in schizophrenia

It would seem, then, that attention to compromises in the dialogical self enriches our understanding of how one can and does experience oneself as diminished. We would now like to suggest that our approach could also offer a new taxonomy of scenarios in which such feelings of diminishment arise. In particular, we find three models of self-organization that both result from compromises in the interanimating flow of self-positions and lead to experiences of self-diminishment.

The monological self

Our first model involves a significant decrease in the interanimating play of self-positions due to the inflexible dominance of one or two self-positions. In such cases, a rigidly unchanging hierarchy emerges in which self–world interactions are consistently ordered in a singular manner, and intra- and interpersonal dialogue is replaced by a monologue. Now, the monologue may prove internally consistent, but its inflexibility leaves one unable to respond to changing situations, resulting in limited action orientations and a compromised basis for shared understanding with others, particularly if one's monologue is built around implausible interpretations of oneself and the world. Moreover, when such a state of affairs is contrasted with one's past, one can only sense one's self as having come apart somewhere along the way.

The cases of Grieg and Frank strike us as clear manifestations of monological self-organization. Both are able to recognize objects and perform basic human actions, but their general sense for the situations in which they find themselves, and thus for the opportunities and challenges they face, is severely limited and inflexible. Frank was formerly a man who loved certain people, rebelled against others, and who had strong passions, e.g., concerning music, and doubts about qualitatively different life possibilities, e.g., his ability to do well at college. After onset, however, his world contracted into a drama of personal persecution. At the beginning of his psychotherapy, Grieg had two different ways in which to respond and experience himself: as someone about to be killed, or as the object of unimaginable praise and affirmation. Before the emergence of these parallel monologues, however, he led a varied life with varied opportunities and challenges. He dreamt of being a carpenter, loved certain people, disliked others, struggled to be a good son, and grieved a lost brother. Yes, these life trajectories might flow into one another, but they had integrity of their own, and that is precisely what disappears when one's life takes a monological turn. A car drives past because Frank is in danger. People at the supermarket gawk because they know that celebrities love Grieg.

When a life take this monological turn, one's sense of self is swallowed up in the singular self-disclosures monologues provide. A survey of Grieg and Frank's discursive self-presentations reveals that genuine interplay among self-positions is noticeably lacking. Certainly, we can form ideas of what Frank and Grieg might be feeling and experiencing, but to gain any concrete impression of who either man is stems from far-reaching inferences that we, the listeners, make about *how* either man speaks rather than from any grasp of *what* either says.

Grieg could only repeat the same general story, again and again, presenting himself as either universally beloved or besieged, with an occasional observation that he simply had become his mental illness. Frank was similarly locked within a recurring story, and when pushed past the confines of his paranoid situation, he only found emptiness, inside and out. But as we've suggested, if sense of self is given in the play of self-positions, this is precisely what one would expect to find. Once a monologue is in force, only one or two themes/ideas fund interpretations of emotions, daily events, and the behavior of others, thereby disclosing one's own being in equally constrained terms. Moreover, such a narrow range of interpretation will eventually strain social relations and weaken one's ability to navigate changing circumstances, thereby compounding one's sense that meaningful agency lies beyond one's reach.

The barren self

A second model of compromised self-organization can be gleaned from the cases of Webern and Glass. Webern, who we have described elsewhere (Lysaker, Buck and Hammoud, 2007), is a man in his thirties with psychiatric symptoms meeting DSM-IV-TR criteria for schizophrenia, undifferentiated subtype. He was one of several siblings born and raised in an intact family, with one of his parents experiencing severe mental illness. He finished high school, worked a series of jobs requiring minimal skills, and became estranged from his family in early adulthood. By his mid-twenties, he was unable to keep a job for more than a matter of weeks. Around this time, he experienced several hospitalizations and faced a variety of legal problems arising from aggressive social behavior. His difficulties evident, he was awarded a disability pension. After being incarcerated for a month in a local jail, he began receiving psychotherapy.

Webern experienced significant delusions and actively responded to auditory hallucinations. He demonstrated flat affect, a paucity of speech and thought, and his motor movements were retarded. He only spoke when addressed, and then offered little. If asked about his emotional state, his prototypical reply was 'fine'. When asked why he came to the clinic, he would say, 'I have schizophrenia.' When asked what that meant, he would state that he was too old for strenuous activity. When asked for his thoughts, he usually would deny having any. When asked how he came to be in legal trouble, he would indicate that he went somewhere too often. When asked where, he would identify it as a hotel. When asked what he did to attract police attention, he would state that he was too old to go there. When asked about his quietness, he would say: 'Forgot how to talk.' When asked whether he once could talk, he would reply 'yes'. When asked if he wanted to relearn to talk, he would say 'sure'. Webern could describe events, but he never linked those events to anything he felt, thought, or did.

Glass is a man in his fifties with a 30-year history of suffering from schizophrenia. Since his twenties, he continuously experienced levels of hallucinations and delusions, which included hearing people cursing him and beliefs that he was followed wherever he went. Intermittently, Glass experienced bizarre ideation and formal thought disorder that resulted in several, relatively brief hospitalizations. He is a lifelong bachelor and has never had difficulties with substance abuse or the law. When he came to us, he was living with a sibling and unemployed, although prior to that, he worked steadily, including a decade of work in a highly technical field.

When asked how the clinic could assist him, Glass described his life as 'being in a cloudbank' and described himself as having 'commit-ment terror'. He noted that he more or less hypothetically knew what he needed to do to improve his life, e.g., find a new job, but he was aware of nothing that interested him. Nevertheless, he blankly explained that he had nothing to say about himself. He was fully aware of how to list goals, prioritize them, and solve problems (e.g., applying for a job or pursuing a relationship), but these thoughts were merely ideas and never coalesced into actions. According to him, he simply could not will himself to do those things. When asked what he made of all of this, he suggested that such things concerned matters that only a doctor would understand. He wasn't depressed; it was simply that he experienced himself as lacking any influence over what was going on in his mind or in the world around him. Moreover, he found it absurd that he should be struggling so much.

On our view, Webern and Glass exemplify another possible outcome for those whose self-positions have ceased to dialogue with one another in meaningful ways. When asked about why his life had the cast it did, Webern repeatedly described himself as too old for strenuous activity. Similarly, Glass presented himself as confused and adrift, a cloudbank, and he was at a loss with regard to how he might change his circum-stances. But things end there. Both remarked that they had no account of themselves, and nothing in what they said has a strong relation to preced-ing or succeeding events. Instead, each statement seemed to exist in isola-tion; it neither contradicted nor complemented what came before.

It is of particular note that Webern and Glass presented themselves in ways that lack even the singular focus (and thus the internal coherence) of monological self-presentations. Instead, it is as if they are ciphers through which disjointed remarks and actions flow. Webern has 'forgotten how to talk'. This may mean that he has something to say, but regardless, the life that he would talk about, namely his, isn't relating to itself in an interanimating manner. Unlike Webern, Glass thinks that he can speak and reason without difficulty, but since he finds nothing that would direct him or bring his thoughts and feelings into action, a similar disjunction between the facets of his life is apparent.

The emptied, disjointed way in which Webern and Glass communicate, and the ways in which they present themselves as lost, too old, or bereft of former abilities evidences a sense that through the course of their illness, each has diminished to a point of bareness, as if they were mere placeholders for events they observe but do not influence. Here self-positions arise, but without any interanimating play. Rather, they unfold down seemingly discrete paths. Therefore, whatever sense of self a given character or organism-position provides will depart once it runs its pre-reflectively charted course, and this will leave one with the sense of being lost in a life run more or less on autopilot. Consistent with Calasso's (1994) description of those who suffer at the hands of Greek gods, these men appear unable to imagine that their thoughts, words, or deeds could influence their fate.

A lack of interanimating play among self-positions has other consequences as well. Under such conditions, the kind of life narrative made possible by communicative competence proves impossible. (We thus find it telling that Webern presents himself as having forgotten how to talk). Moreover, meta-positions that reflect who we think we're becoming will never arise, thus offering nothing to fill the gap left in the wake of departing character and organism-positions. (At least the monological type is afforded a meta-position, deluded as it is).

Finally, limited to more or less entrenched self-positions whose relations and relative standing do not change, people like Webern and Glass fare poorly in a world that both involves swiftly changing interpersonal landscapes and requires extensive planning as well as ongoing presentations of what one has done and where one is going. We note this because aggravated social relationships only compound feelings of powerlessness and loss, thus intensifying the sense that one has some-how become unmoored and diminished as a meaningful and effective presence in the world and in one's life.

The cacophonous self

Thus far we've presented two models of self-organization in which breakdowns in intra- and interpersonal dialogue lead to a sense of one-self as diminishing. We now turn to a third model, the cacophonous self, in which certain people suffering from schizophrenia find them-selves in a swirl of self-positions that seems to proceed without any order at all.

Consider the case of Purcell, whom we have also described elsewhere (Lysaker and Lysaker, 2006). Purcell is a man in his forties with schizo-phrenia, disorganized subtype. At the onset of his psychotherapy, his speech was loud and rapid with frequent loose associations and occa-sional neologisms. His affect ranged from blunted to inappropriate, with occasional, poorly modulated explosions of anxiety and fear that seemed unrelated to the environment. He believed that others could enter his body and cause him pain, noted that he heard voices around him, and believed that he was persecuted by an 'other' who seemed to be everyone around him. He had experienced over 20 years of institutionalization where he received what appeared to be custodial care. For that period of time, he reported having no close friends, steady unemployment, and continuous alienation from family. He had a history of childhood sexual trauma and a host of legal problems in adolescence and adulthood. Physically, he was in poor health and suf-fered from chronic pain. Neurocognitive testing indicated profound deficits in verbal memory and executive function. He came to psy-chotherapy following a transfer from a long-term inpatient unit to a group home which was necessitated by the inpatient unit's diminishing resources.

When Purcell spoke about past and present mundane events, it was nearly impossible to follow him. Events were rarely temporally sequenced and the people involved were almost never mentioned by name. Because it is so hard to describe how such speech proceeds, permit us two examples:

> Because it's hard finding yourself again. Anybody can come up with a question and turn the whole picture around. Anybody can find an answer and they can't stand you. But if you got something to hold, that you can hold against them, that'll tear you to pieces and tear them to pieces. And somebody may be sticking up for your life on one side, and on the other side it may be your own family. They don't want them to take your part.

He continues:

> I went absent without giving notice a few times from the service while I was in there. I don't know why ... it was my fault, because either way if I didn't go absent without leave, if I stayed in there I was in great danger. I already had something wrong with me, accidents that were inflicted and accidental, and in ways of life I had a challenge because there was a great opportunity going on then by surrounding companies and stuff. A person can make a living outside the company and don't have to work for the company, which is bad in one sense and good on the other sense. This is mixed up, but I can't align the stories straight because they're all different time frames.

Drawing from the terms we have developed, it appears that Purcell's intra- and interpersonal dialogues have entered a state of cacophony. He can speak, and expressively so (there is palpable pain in the first excerpt), but his remarks are cryptic. Individual statements seem marginally related to those that precede and follow them. The second excerpt loses its narrative thread amid shifting dramatic scenes (the service, surrounding companies, work outside a particular company) and shifting temporal registers. Moreover, each scene involves apparently distinct character-positions, namely, self-as-soldier and self-as-worker, which are never brought into conversation with one another. To the degree this excerpt has an overarching theme, it involves a series of morally confusing situations. These observations, which could potentially lead to the articulation of a meta-position, bubble up from within each scene rather than order them for the purpose of making a general point. In the first excerpt, there is an overall tone of conflict, even frustration, but no definite dramatic center. Yes, Purcell begins with the task of 'finding yourself again', but it fails to effectively order the events that follow: people asking questions, those who find answers but who 'can't stand' Purcell, and somebody supporting Purcell while his family opposed that support.

In Purcell's self-presentations, we find little sense of a person carrying out a life of his or her choosing. In fact, very little beyond pain and confusion emerges, and so one is hard pressed to find among his remarks an individual with articulated hopes and dreams experiencing varied and determinate associations, opportunities, and challenges. Even his pain is something Purcell's speech manifests rather than articulates. In this regard, he manifests a fate similar to what we found in the barrenness of Glass and Webern's self-presentations, but unlike Webern and Glass, his dilemma does not entail minimally articulated, discrete scenarios. Instead, he is caught up in a whirl of associations and disjunctions, a nearly surreal surfeit of self–world interactions and self-presentations, rather than a sparsely dotted landscape.

In a heart-rending way, the first excerpt indirectly articulates Purcell's existential situation. He is unable to find himself again, suggesting that he now senses himself in a state of diminishment. Moreover, whatever he finds can be turned around at the drop of a question, which suggests that his sense of self is quite tenuous at this point. Even more tellingly, the first excerpt suggests that even the search is subject to interruption and redirection. It begins with the question of finding yourself but ends with an amorphous reference to some struggle between Purcell's family and an advocate of his. Purcell thus not only experiences himself as tenuously present in the course of his life, but his efforts to address this lack, even under therapeutic conditions, are undone in what appears as a disordered play of memories, affects, and barely determined self-positions.

In his cacophony, Purcell exemplifies a third model of self-organization that we associate with schizophrenia. Moreover, we think that it too follows from disrupted, interanimating plays among self-positions. If almost no order were present amid intra- and interpersonal dialogues, then one would expect a disorienting play of self-positions and the psychic life they help anchor. With various self-positions appearing and receding without evident order, which means that the various self–world scenarios to which they are tied would appear in kind, one would expect confusion and a series of disjointed reports. Self-positions might briefly come to the fore, but amid rapidly switching self-positions and self–world locations, a determined sense of where one was, with whom, and where one was heading would be hard to come by. The indeterminate scenes that Purcell presents are thus in keeping with one whose points of self–world interaction are so unstable. Finally, amid the turbulence, sense of self would prove equally disoriented. Without a determinate and ordered set of pursuits to reflect upon, pursuits involving character and organism-positions, meta-positions would be very difficult to generate. Likewise, the sense of self that accompanies character and organism-positions would also be fleeting and unstable. Not that these positions disappear altogether in cases like Purcell's. Rather, their ability to disclose a self to itself would be severely compromised if the course of their appearance and recession were frequently interrupted. Such a dialogue would be more akin to a large group of people all speaking at once.

Whereas monological self-organizations seem to cripple one with an inflexible and suffocating order, cacophonous self-organizations push one to the brink of incoherence, tugging a bit at the very logic of a sense of self. Amid cacophony, any X that one might find oneself being seems too unstable to affect the kind of disclosure that gives one a sense of self. Yet Purcell's self-presentation manifests all too clearly a sense of being overwhelmed, even if this sense lacks the meta-positional explicitness that defines monological self-organizations. It thus makes sense to articulate a third pattern of self-organization that arises in schizophrenia. It involves profound disruptions in the interanimating flow of self-positions and leads to experiences of one's self as diminished.

Summary

This chapter has attempted to demonstrate that significantly compromised intra- and interpersonal dialogues can help explain the experience of self-diminishment that often accompanies the appearance of schizophrenia. Such an account is useful because it both clarifies and helps explain a neglected facet of schizophrenia, and in a manner that preserves the first-person dimensions of the illness. Moreover, it does so in a way that helps synthesize observations from diverse theoretical perspectives. Second, we have presented three models of

Table 4.1 Three forms of diminished self-experience

Model	Description	Examples
Monological	an inflexible dominance of one or two meta-positions, which leads to implausible interpretations of self and world, and a repetitive life-narrative	Frank's fear that everything he experiences belongs to a plot to kill him
Barren	undeveloped, mostly discontinuous self-positions, which lead to a fragmented life-narrative populated by few meta-positions and limited descriptions of the world	Glass's sense of being adrift in a 'cloudbank' and unable to change his circumstances
Cacophonous	an often rapid and chaotic succession of self-positions, which leads to an incoherent life-narrative filled with abstract generalizations	Purcell's cryptic and temporally jumbled self-presentations

dialogical compromise that lead to experiences of self-diminishment. These are gathered in Table 4.1.

We consider these models useful additions to the literature because they refine our feel for what it is like to undergo schizophrenia, and they help us distinguish some markedly different ways in which someone's sense of self can be undermined over the course of the illness.

Chapter 5

Dialogical compromise and symptoms

In the last chapter we suggested that experiences of diminished subjectivity in schizophrenia could be clarified and accounted for in part by disruptions in dialogical processes. If interanimating play among self-positions falls into disorder, dialogical processes will no longer be able to constitute and sustain an evolving self-experience, which in turn could lead people to regard themselves as diminished or on the verge of destruction. Disorder of this kind does not fully undermine one's ability to sense one's self, however, and thus approaching experiences of self-disruption through dialogical compromise could also account for how people, such as those who have schizophrenia, can experience their own diminishment. We additionally suggested that a dialogical account of self-disruption in schizophrenia might advance our understanding of the varieties of self-disruption. In particular, we suggested that breakdowns in the play of self-positions likely result in the emergence of one or more analytically distinct types of disrupted self-experience: a cacophony, a barren and empty landscape, and a monologue where intra- and inter-personal polyphony is dominated by and withers under a single view.

While our view may begin to account for some of the more puzzling subjective aspects of schizophrenia, how does it bear upon objective signs and symptoms? Are there implications here for understanding schizophrenia's classic features? Or have we run into a dualism involving an ill mind, understood in terms of a compromised sense of self, and an ill brain, understood in terms of symptoms? We suggest that recuperating the first-person dimensions of schizophrenia does not institute yet another version of mind–body dualism. Central to our view is the claim that one can fruitfully integrate the so-called 'objective' and 'subjective' aspects of schizophrenia into a more unified theory. Accordingly, this chapter will explore the relevance of dialogical processes for an understanding of five symptoms drawn from three of the broad classes of traditional symptoms associated with schizophrenia. Specifically, we will examine how dialogical disruptions could be influenced by and exert influence over complex verbal hallucinations, systematized delusions, blunted affect, lack of volition, and unawareness of illness.

A final observation before proceeding. We do not believe that self-experience in schizophrenia can be reduced to the traditional symptoms under consideration here. Nor do we think that the symptoms are merely a disguised form of altered self-experience. There are a number of non-psychiatric conditions in which symptoms similar to those in schizophrenia may occur without the same changes in subjective experience. For instance, people suffering from Alzheimer's, a head injury or stroke can experience symptoms similar to those of schizophrenia without an analogous subjective perception of self-destruction. Similarly, people who experience hallucinations or who embrace any number of unusual, socially non-validated convictions but do not have a medical condition can nevertheless have a strong, coherent sense of self (Leudar and Thomas, 2000). Our claim, then, is that distinct phenomena can contribute to the course of schizophrenia, and in manners that mutually influence, even build upon one another.

Dialogical disruption and two forms of positive symptoms

Complex verbal hallucinations

Positive symptoms, as noted in Chapter 1, reflect the intrusion of uncommon experiences into consciousness. The first type we will discuss is complex verbal hallucinations. Hallucinations involve either a false sensory experience or mistaking a mental phenomenon for a sensory one of any modality. Hearing a voice no one can hear, smelling a foul odor, feeling insects crawling under one's skin, seeing a vision of a devil, seeing colors in the sky, hearing thunder when there is none, or hearing God are all examples of hallucinations that could occur in schizophrenia.

Complex verbal hallucinations refer to one specific form of hallucination. They are auditory hallucinations in which one not only hears a voice, but it relays a coherent message or command. So, hearing indistinct voices whispering would not be a complex verbal hallucination. Nor would hearing nonsense syllables or someone calling your name. Grieg, however, whom we discussed in Chapter 4, experienced complex verbal hallucinations. He heard the voices of celebrities on television praising his masculinity. He sat alone in his living room and heard a detailed commentary on his special abilities, which he believed emanated from his television.

To date, systematic surveys suggest that complex hallucinations are common in acute (Benjamin, 1989) and post-acute (Nayani and David, 1996) phases of schizophrenia. It has also been frequently reported that these voices express a wish or intention to regulate or influence the behavior of the person hearing them, and that these sources are experienced as omnipotent (Birchwood *et al.*, 2000; Chadwick and Birchwood, 1994; Davies *et al.*, 1999; Leudar and Thomas, 2000). Gilbert and colleagues (2001) have suggested that, beyond causing an individual to engage in specific behaviors, hallucinations may also trigger basic human responses, e.g., an immediate inclination to flee or aggress.

As will become evident, it is of particular interest to us that complex hallucinations tend to communicate focused, singular messages. Grieg heard voices telling him that he possessed masculine qualities, which surpassed those of all the men around him, but that is all they said. It is also noteworthy that complex verbal hallucinations do not invite the hearer to reply. In a complex verbal hallucination, a person may fear, loathe, love, or hate the voice uttering the complex message. They also may debate with themselves or others about the meaning of the voice's message (e.g., Benjamin, 1989; Davies *et al.*, 1999; Leudar and Thomas, 2000). The individual may even shout at the voice or distract themselves from its insistent proclamation, but the voice is generally not construed as something one can talk with or influence. Grieg does not speak back to the celebrities praising him. The address is purely unidirectional, and he does not experience these voices as open to influence from anything he might say or do. Instead, they are somewhat analogous to a god or a military commander with whom it is inappropriate to converse. Most generally, then, Grieg experienced his hallucinations as unidirectional proclamations urging him to act and/or feel in a certain way.

Whether complex verbal hallucinations have their root in abnormal spontaneous cortical activity in centers that support language (David, 1994), or in any other source, their place in dialogical processes seems discernable. First, in the presence of complex verbal hallucinations, intrapersonal dialogue should suffer constant interruptions. Just as anyone finds it difficult to think and function in the presence of comments that issue orders or arouse fight or flight responses, it would seem that movement among self-positions would proceed tentatively at best when one undergoes complex verbal hallucinations. In fact, one might find oneself in the organism-position that arises with fight or flight responses. At least, the action orientations that commence with character-positions would meet with great resistance, particularly if one's hallucinations arrived with absolute authority.

Our suggestion, then, is that as complex verbal hallucinations gain strength in schizophrenia, a person's usual dialogical movements are likely to be interrupted and colonized by the monologue delivered by the hallucination. Grieg, by his own account, could spend hours listening to voices address him, thinking of little else. From the complementary perspective of his therapist, it seemed that the voices provided a monologue that he could not question and which subsumed his identity. It would seem, then, that complex verbal hallucinations could corrode dialogical processes and therefore affect experiences of diminishment.

Perhaps, though, the voices that people like Grieg hear create a chorus that commences a new dialogue even as it disrupts existing ones. Might not the voices of celebrities that seemed to address Grieg provide a field for possible dialogue? Without excluding the possibility, we think not. Since interaction with voices is unidirectional, it is unlikely that Grieg found room for dialogue with his insistent admirers. Of course, it may be possible that voices remind people of self-facets, which then initiate an interanimating play, but in order for that play to sustain itself, the monological presence of complex verbal hallucinations will have to slacken significantly. Remember, multiple self-positions can appear in monological self-organizations, but interanimating dialogue is then suppressed as the recurrent story reasserts itself.

Even noting their disruptive influence, it is difficult to ignore the likelihood that Grieg's hallucinations protected him from two different kinds of threats: the threat of any view of himself as totally inadequate, as well as the threat that his self-organization would deteriorate into a generally cacophonous state. By providing him with a meta-position, namely, self-as-important, Grieg's hallucinations soothed and organized his self-experience even as they left him a passive recipient of his own life direction. We do think, therefore, that some hallucinations, while momentarily compromising the capacity for dialogue, may help sustain a meta-positional sense of self that might later be enlivened in and even sustain dialogue. Indeed, in our later chapter on psychotherapy, it will be observed that this sense of self as valued by others could be awakened and tied to others in a dialogical manner.

Dialogical processes and systematized delusions

A second kind of positive symptom that may be linked to alterations in self-experience is systematized delusion. Delusions, as described in the first chapter, involve thoughts that others in one's community find extremely implausible. This is not to say, however, that the views of one culture or subculture that another considers implausible are delusional. For instance, a view shared across one's church that the world will end on a certain date would not be a delusion, even if this view is not shared by other religions. We should also point out that false beliefs are not delusional. Intensely believing that one's spouse is having an affair would not necessarily be a delusion, even if false. The issue lies in part with plausibility, or rather, one's appreciation for the plausibility of one's thought, and so thinking that one's spouse is having an affair with an alien from outer space would be a delusion.[1]

As in the case of hallucinations, there are many forms of delusions. People may believe a stone has taken the place of their heart, that they are dead, can walk through walls, or stop the rain. They may insist that they are an incarnation of a Tibetan spirit, or that large networks of people are watching them for reasons they cannot uncover. Systematized delusions are unusually stable, and they explain and link together a wide range of potentially unrelated events according to one or a limited number of themes. Like complex verbal hallucinations, they incline a person to view the world in a singular manner, and they do not appear to be matters for dialogue, reflection, or inquiry.

Systematic delusions form an unassailable starting point around which a life revolves. A sense that people are watching whenever one leaves home would not be a systematized delusion. Repeatedly entertaining the thought that a man in Ann Arbor, Michigan with ties to the United Nations, winemakers in California, and the CIA are monitoring one's every move in order to ascend to power would be a systematized delusion. As detailed in a previous chapter, Frank suffered from systematized delusion. He was convinced graffiti exposed his embarrassing sexual practices. Moreover, he thought the graffiti, as well as the movement of cars outside his parents' home involved people organized by someone plotting to kill him, namely, the spouse of a former teacher.

Because of their non-negotiable authority, systematized delusions strain an individual's abilities to sustain diverse intra- and interpersonal dialogue, thereby contributing to a diminished sense of self. Once in place, systematized delusions will likely institute a monological self-organization, which trumps the action orientations and self-disclosures of one's character and meta-positions. Consider Frank's absolute certainty about the plot hatched to kill him. When his delusion was active, Frank's dialogical processes contracted to a meta-position like 'self-as-persecuted', with a possible corresponding organism-position flush with panic. As Frank himself explained, the omnipresence of the plot to kill him brought about only two emotions, rage and panic, and they overrode whatever other self-positions might emerge. In other words, in the midst of his delusions, Frank only had two voices or self-positions with which to address himself and others. As we've noted, when he stopped thinking about his persecution, he was equally overwhelmed by a sense of nothingness and pain. Thus, as in the case of complex verbal hallucinations, systematized delusions also seem to corrode dialogical processes and amplify experiences of self-diminishment.

Can delusions sustain a failing dialogue? We would again suggest that this is unlikely. In their acute phases, delusions undermine the interanimating play of self-positions that is the essence of the dialogical self. However, lurking within the meta-position 'self-as-persecuted', one might find evidence of being a very important person of great interest to many in power. In an indirect and complex manner, then, it is possible that such beliefs provide a minimally positive sense of self amid profound diminishment, and in a manner that might contribute to rehabilitation somewhere down the road.

Mutual impact in positive symptoms and dialogical compromise

Thus far, we've suggested that complex verbal hallucinations and systematized delusions generally hinder the richness and diversity of intrapersonal dialogue, thereby contributing to experiences of diminishing subjectivity in schizophrenia. Before we consider other symptoms, we also wish to suggest that positive symptoms and disrupted dialogical processes could mutually influence one another, developing momentum as distinct self-positions are absorbed. At base, our claim is that as positive symptoms imperil dialogue, disruptions in intrapersonal dialogue heighten positive symptoms. With fewer self-positions available, the singular, impelling voice of a complex hallucination or systematized delusion should gain strength. If one has few voices within oneself, it might prove increasingly difficult not to follow and be defined by one's symptoms.

In order to detail our suggestion, let's construe some general, hypothetical examples. Suppose that character-positions like self-as-student and self-as-son are colonized by a monological self-organization. As the action trajectories of character-positions are interrupted, the sense of self they provide departs as well, leaving one with fewer points from which to call into question the reality or authority of the voices one hears. If the result is a more or less monological self-organization, then each self–world interaction will reinforce the presence of the delusion or the authority of the story line demanded by one's complex verbal hallucinations. Moreover, the social relationships anchored in part by one's character-positions will suffer as well, thereby intensifying feelings of social alienation and stress. This in turn will intensify experiences of diminishment and possibly undermine the force of meta-positions, e.g., self-as-critical or self-as-level-headed, that might enable one to resist the pull of one's delusions. This latter result seems very probable if one's sense of self becomes dominated by a monologically generated meta-position. Under these conditions, reflection only ever finds the force of one's delusions or the orientation, for example, self-as-savior, provided by one's hallucinations.

On the whole, then, our hypothesis is that with fewer self-positions available, it becomes increasingly difficult to reject delusions or hallucinations. One will have difficulty saying 'that is not me', 'that is very unlikely', or 'that is not the kind of person I am', and so one's symptoms may intensify and/or assume a greater role in one's self-organization. If this is right, then, in the intersection of positive symptoms and dialogical processes, mutual influence can be found. Positive symptoms seem to undermine the interanimating interplay of self-positions, even as decrements in dialogical capacity, and thereby sense of self, seem to heighten vulnerability to the influence of positive symptoms.

We find it important to acknowledge the interplay of positive symptoms and declining dialogical capacities because it helps us understand cases like Grieg's, which involve the slow erosion of a life amid a gradual amplification of symptoms. We have suggested that while Grieg once experienced a rich series of intra- and interpersonal exchanges, they fell away over time. Self-as-son-who-disappointed-the-mother, self-as-lover-of-wife, self-as-unappreciated-worker, self-as-grateful-father, self-as-loved-by-brother, and self-as-future-carpenter were replaced over the years by a relatively small number of self-positions that seemed unconnected to concrete life situations and lacked the presence of determinate others.

Viewed from the third-person, Grieg's contracting dialogical processes and corresponding sense of gradual diminishment seems clearly entwined with the development of his symptoms. In fact, none of his illness's dimensions seem anything more than analytically distinct since dialogical atrophy and his experiences of diminishment went hand in hand with an increased presence of hallucinatory experiences and/or delusional beliefs. Said otherwise, Grieg's case does not present a simple, linear chain of cause and effect. Rather, the emergence of symptoms, the corrosion of dialogical capacity, and experiences of self-diminishment seem to unfold in mutually intensifying, recursive processes. Regarding this as a likely state of affairs proves easier, we think, if we consider Grieg's fate over the 20-year period that followed the onset of his illness. Seen as a whole, it is not hard to imagine how weakening dialogical capacities made it harder for him to make sense of, or ward off, extremely anomalous experiences, including implausible beliefs and sensory experiences not shared by others. Further, the more the experience of psychosis intruded into his psyche, the more we might expect his intra- and interpersonal dialogues to wither, all leading to greater and greater levels of social alienation. With fewer people to speak with, with greater losses to make sense of, and with fewer cognitive resources, we can imagine that it gradually became easier and easier for Grieg to interpret the world in terms of his persecution by nameless forces or his high standing with celebrities, despite the fact that these explanations were exceedingly far-fetched, lacked any genuine evidence, and made it increasingly difficult to manage the dilemmas of daily life. Finally, alone and with little to say about himself that either concretely addressed or could be acknowledged by others, one could see why he gradually came to regard himself as simply an instance of his mental illness.

On our view, finding himself lost in his mental illness was not simply a conclusion that Grieg drew from the presence of his symptoms. Rather, our claim is that with the arrival of symptoms, he experienced an increasing sense of diminishment amid dialogical disruption which reduced his capacity to stave off symptoms. This then fed back into his reduced dialogical capacity, which weakened social capacity and undermined social ties, all feeding back into a vicious circle whereby self-disturbance and psychopathology sustained and supported one another. In other words, in cases like Grieg's, it appears that the way in which he experienced and underwent his illness was a constitutive part of the illness, not simply a subjective awareness of so-called objective events.

Dialogical disruption and two forms of negative symptoms

Blunted affect and the dialogical self

While positive symptoms entail the presence of unexpected sensory experiences or implausible thoughts, negative symptoms, as detailed in the first chapter, suggest an absence of experiences one usually expects. This can include a paucity of feelings, desires, gestures, words, or a lack of drive and persistence that commonly characterize people's lives. The prevailing view is that negative symptoms have unique etiological roots. Someone with schizophrenia can have both positive and negative symptoms, just positive, or just negative symptoms, but it has been suggested that distinct neuropathologies underlie each class (e.g., Andreasen *et al.*, 1990).

The first type of negative symptom we'd like to discuss is blunted affect, which generally refers to a lack of emotional expression in inflection, expression, and gesture. A person described as having blunted affect would show a limited range of emotion, perhaps appearing wooden or lifeless in the midst of a celebration or a time of sadness. In contrast to a depressed person who might silently be consumed by pain, someone with flat affect would feel emptiness. If confronted with something painful, pleasurable, surprising, or disgusting, a person with flat affect would show the same emotional response: nothing. Again, he or she wouldn't be sadly disinterested or mournfully aloof. Rather, the experience of a negative symptom is the experience of an absence. Someone with lack of or flattened affect feels close to nothing in contexts where one would expect some degree of emotional response.

Both Glass and Webern, whom we discussed in Chapter 4, appear to experience blunted affect. Glass tells us that he is in a cloudbank, suggesting a hazy, undifferentiated state within which direction is elusive. Moreover, none of the events wherein his life unfolds produces any particular effect in him, as if each self–world interaction were just more mist and vapor, including his own role therein. While he has plenty of ideas about what he might do, none stir him to excitement or worry. He can cognitively articulate a future, but he does so without affect.

In fact, whenever asked about what he feels, he says nothing and intimates that therapists should know the feelings of people like him, i.e., those with severe mental illness. Moreover, while saying this, he sits calmly, makes few gestures, and speaks with very little inflection in his voice.

Webern, perhaps even more so than Glass, shows no emotion, even when discussing things related to him. He lacks inflection when he speaks to the point that he sounds like a robot in a science fiction movie, and his facial expression does not change. When questioned about his demeanor, he says that he has forgotten how to talk, which we take to mean that he has forgotten how to express himself. Not unexpectedly, when asked, he denies that he feels pain. He says he is 'fine' in response to all inquiries but also admits that this is his answer to everything. One time, when pressed to admit that seeing a probation officer was unpleasant, he initially said, 'No, it was fine.' When asked if most people would be upset in such a situation, he said, 'Of course', but he neither responded to nor drew any consequences from this discrepancy. Like Glass, he seems adrift and disconnected from his life. He once recalled watching a basketball game and he described it as fine, but he could not name the teams playing or recall the score. When asked if that were strange, he said, 'It's fine,' but, yes, it struck him as 'strange'; he used to 'know what was happening around him'.

On our view, negative symptoms, like positive symptoms, could disrupt intrapersonal dialogue, leading to experiences of self-diminishment. Regardless of the etiology of blunted affect, when a person experiences a decrease in available affect, it seems likely that the strength of certain self-positions could erode, disrupting the capacity to play various social roles. Consider again the different facets of Raskolnikov, the main character in *Crime and Punishment*. Dostoyevsky tells us that he is '... sullen, gloomy, arrogant, proud ... insecure ... magnanimous and kind ... cold and callous ... always in a hurry, always too busy and lies there doing nothing'. As self-positions, these strike us as a series of meta-positions, directly tied to affect, which describe how Raskolnikov conducts himself, or carries out his many character-positions. Suppose that he were beset by blunted affect. Could he still behave in a manner that is sullen, proud, or insecure? Evidently not, for each of these moods suggests a concerned response to the world, and this is precisely what blunted affect undermines. So, should blunted affect enter Raskolnikov's self-organization, these meta-positions would prove increasingly unrecognizable, and as they linger, they only would enter the interanimating flow of self-positions as memorials of who he once had been, thus contributing to a sense of self as diminished.

Not only meta-positions would be threatened by blunted affect, however. Recall that meta-positions reflect ways in which one experiences and interprets one's conduct as manifest in character and organism-positions. If those ways of carrying oneself fade, what will animate one's character-positions? How will one conduct roles like friend, worker, citizen, etc.? The question has force because intra- and inter-personal dialogue is an interanimating process, and so, should animation wane in a general way, dialogue might largely come to a halt. Blunted affect seems to lead in this direction. Just as 'self-as-activist' will fade as a character-position if one becomes increasingly apathetic, so too will the full range of one's character-positions contract if one's overall affect dissipates. Yes, their action orientations may persist in outline, e.g., Webern seems to still know how to watch a basketball game, but those performances don't really expand into rich, distinct self–world orientations capable of either manifesting the diversity of one's being or attending to the diversity of the world. It is thus unsurprising that Webern repeatedly announces that he is 'fine'. It's as if 'self-as-fine' is a persistent organism-position. His overall state was neither good nor bad – just fine. Not that he found equanimity. Rather, it's as if he's just barely there, and always in more or less the same way, which leaves him aware that he has lost the person he once was, as well as the world that once 'happened around him'.

As with complex verbal hallucinations and systematized delusions, it seems that one can make the case that systematized blunted affect erodes the interanimating flow of self-positions. In this case, however, the disruption results from the loss of animating force as opposed to the stark interruption of competing voices. Regardless, in stalling the play of self-positions that provides one with a sense of self, persistently blunted affect still contributes to the sense that one has somehow diminished.

Negative symptoms: lack of volition and its impact on the dialogical self

The second negative symptom we'd like to discuss concerns distur-bances in or the absence of volition. Whereas someone suffering from blunted affect responds to self–world interactions in flat, emotionless ways, someone experiencing a disturbance of volition is unable to initi-ate goal-directed activity or make purposeful decisions. It isn't that he or she is ambivalent or torn between two desirable or undesirable alternatives. Nor is he or she in too much pain to act. Rather, some-thing is missing – that which we metaphorically term 'will power'. Consequently, people suffering from lack of volition do nothing from day to day. They are simply not compelled to pursue any particular course of action.

Glass seems to suffer from this symptom. He has thoughts about what he could do, even 'should' do, but nothing impels him to action. His musings on his future are thus just that, a kind of idle speculation. Webern's case is similar but his lack of volition seems more profound. He observes his life, but only that. In fact, he finds it beyond the bounds of possibility that he might initiate something and change his circumstances. He isn't paralyzed by pain or uncertainty; he just doesn't initiate action with any deliberate, let alone long-range, intent or purpose. He can attend appointments because 'they tell me' to do so. He eats 'whatever they serve' at his dormitory. He watches 'whatever they put on television'. His self–world interactions are thus remarkably passive, as if he were internalizing external directives at every turn.

In our view, profoundly diminished volition can negatively impact sense of self. Character-positions provide a sense of self through their action orientations, which are directed towards determinate ends. Sense of self primarily arises, however, through the actualization of these orientations. For example, being a student is in large part a matter of doing the things that students do, such as attending class, doing homework, and learning, and in a manner oriented towards the ends associated with education, for example, edification and/or improved employment opportunities. However, if one only ever follows the most basic and minimal rules associated with a particular role, for example, going where one is told to go, eating what one is told to eat, watching what one is told to watch, very little of oneself will appear in the course of one's performances. This means, then, that one's character-positions won't provide a very concrete sense of self. Moreover, as they unfold, one's performances will provide little material for meta-positions, which mainly reflect how well one is faring in one's pursuits. In fact, to the degree that one had previously pursued anything at all, under these conditions, current self–world interactions will probably provide evidence contrary to one's previous meta-positions, even if they presented one as a failure. One can't fail if one never pursues anything.

Lack of volition may also slow and frustrate interanimating play among self-positions, which will intensify experiences which suggest that one has diminished. On the one hand, volitional deficits would seem to decrease the number of self-positions at work in one's self-organization, which would diminish the richness of one's pre-reflectively operative, intra- and interpersonal dialogues. As we've just noted, such deficits are likely to shrink the number of meta-positions one has, which would leave one with little to say about one's welfare. Second, without the commitment to perform them in earnest, character-positions not provided by institutional situations will fall to the wayside. If one doesn't do the things associated with being a student, that character-position will cease to be a meaningful voice in one's intra- and interpersonal dialogue, and so the breadth of one's dialogical nature will contract, giving one the sense of having become something less than one formerly was.

Lacking determinate goals also seems to render the activity of narrating one's life story more or less meaningless. Normally we narrate a life story because we find ourselves in a character-position that requires us to account for ourselves. Suppose we're out for dinner, and our date says: 'Tell me about yourself.' Or, suppose you apply for a job, and you're asked to both assemble your employment history and explain why you're making this career move now. In these cases, purposive action, pursued within character-positions, prompts a reflective moment. If one never dates or seeks new employment, however, one has no reason to reflect in these ways, and if one never really pursues anything, then one will simply bypass the kind of reflective dialogue that enables one to reflect on the ensemble one is, formulate meta-positions, and consider new registers for one's unfolding future.

If we think about Webern and Glass in this context, it proves less surprising that neither has very much to say. Glass feels trapped and can object to his fate, but he seeks an external force to speak for him. It is up to the therapist to know his story and what he should be impelled to do. In a similar manner, Webern complies with the events that unfold around him. He can agree with others and describe events, but nothing more. His actions, as they are disclosed to him, don't seem to participate in a larger project that he regards as *his* life. It is as if both men have vanished as agents from the scene of their lives even while they continue to observe that scene and their own diminishing part within it.[2]

Note that we are not claiming that lack of volition leads to the loss of all intra- and interpersonal dialogue. Rather, our claim is that such conditions reduce dialogue to the animation of relatively insular self-positions associated with either subsistence needs or institutional placements secured by others. Moreover, we are suggesting that people in such a state will produce very few, if any meta-positions, and have little to say about themselves or their experiences. In fact, they might turn such matters over to others, or limit their self-presentations to superficial accounts, claiming, like Webern, 'I'm fine', even when led to acknowledge that others in a similar position would not be fine. One would thus expect to find such people sensing, as Glass and Webern do, that they had fundamentally changed, that their world made less sense, and that they no longer did the things they used to do, or much at all for that matter.

Mutual effects of negative symptoms and dialogical compromise upon one another

In this section, we have attempted to illustrate how the absence of affect and volition could severely lessen the diversity and richness of intrapersonal dialogue. Whereas positive symptoms seem to interrupt and/or colonize dialogical processes, negative symptoms seem to erode their momentum and isolate their various moments. With regard to sense of self, the result is much the same, however. As symptoms intensify, the interanimating play among self-positions is disrupted, and experiences of self-diminishment occur. Is this a two-way street, however? In the case of positive symptoms, we suggested that dialogical breakdown and experiences of self-diminishment could feed back into the play of symptoms, intensifying their presence and role in self-organization. We think that negative symptoms unfold in a similar manner, though here losses of character and meta-positions deprive one of opportunities that often invigorate and inspire human action, irrespective of one's momentary demeanor and outlook.

Recall that character-positions primarily operate along habitual lines. They provide, therefore, pre-reflective sources of action. Think of the English phrase 'I could do this in my sleep.' It suggests that certain roles can be played on autopilot. Moreover, in playing them, habitual roles (i.e., self–world interactions) often generate new energy and affect along the way. We recall the point because, if it is true, then the loss of character-positions would entail the loss of opportunities to add intensity and affective depth to our self–world interactions, particularly during periods of low enthusiasm and/or energy for certain practices (or the demands of life in general). In a different way, affirmative meta-positions (e.g., self-as-success, self-as-go-getter, or self-as-hard-worker), also can buoy us during times of ebb. In order to live up to our own self-conceptions, we often persevere at times when the spirit is weak. Should we find ourselves without meta-positions of this sort, we thus will lack this path out of possibly paralyzing doldrums.

As we've seen, the appearance of negative symptoms can result in an eventual decrease in the number of one's character-positions. Such symptoms also can erode the conditions that prompt the emergence of meta-positions. It would seem likely, therefore, that negative symptoms would produce conditions that intensify their own presence and influence in a given self-organization. Consider the cases of Glass and Webern. Both experience little affect in their self–world interactions, which undermines their performance of character-positions. And without the ongoing performance of those positions, they lose the interanimating opportunities that human action provides, opportunities that most folk need to remain committed to and engaged in the projects of their lives. On our view, then, loss of character-positions can work in tandem with diminished affect to leave one feeling trapped in an affectless cloudbank, to use Glass's language. Similarly, with the loss of meta-positions, and without the emergence of new ones, one might, like Webern, remain 'fine', but only fine (in the sense of neither good nor bad). That is, if one's meta-positional sense of self is broadly affectless and incapable of stirring one to action, then present experiences of affectless, volitional paralysis should eventually prove to be self-fulfilling prophecies.

The disruption of self-experience and lack of awareness of illness

Lack of insight and its impact on the dialogical self

A final, intriguing feature of schizophrenia, one possibly linked to changes in dialogical processes is lack of insight into or awareness of illness. While not a diagnostic feature of schizophrenia, between a third to two-thirds of those with this condition deny or are not aware that they have a mental illness (Amador *et al.*, 1994). They may dispute the claim that the experiences they have, which others term hallucinations and/or delusions, are symptoms of a mental illness, even as they more or less successfully interpret other features of their environment. In fact, they may regard similar thoughts and experiences in others as delusions and/or hallucinations, but deny that their experiences and beliefs indicate the presence of mental illness (Startup, 1997). Such denials also have practical corollaries. Alongside denying that they are ill, these people may appear baffled when others suggest that they have an illness, and they often reject well-intentioned advice and help from family and friends.

Grieg, for instance, could acknowledge that he was in a state of distress. Yet he did not think that he had schizophrenia. Grieg knew he heard a voice others did not hear. He also thought that those in his housing project who also heard voices that no one else heard were 'sick in the head'. He also noted problems with 'some depression' and 'too much medication', and he said that his life was not how he would like it to be, but not because he has a mental illness. As to why he did not work, he explained that he would not work for a low wage. Similarly, neither Webern nor Purcell thought that he had a mental illness. For Webern, nothing was wrong, and for Purcell, he was a victim of 'the man' who had 'forced me into a cage'. In his mind, 'society and America' were to blame for his fate. Both agreed to take medicine, but only because they were 'told to'. Purcell knew that pain could enter his body if others wished it to, and Webern knew that he no longer knew how to talk, but again, for neither man did this indicate the presence of a mental illness.

Lack of insight raises problems for treatment.[3] Most models of help-seeking behavior (e.g., Pescosolido, 1997) are based on the core assumption that people who deny that they are ill may neither seek nor accept assistance from others. If this assumption is right, then people who are unaware of their illness may risk prolonged and possibly catastrophic deficits and difficulties. Indeed, research suggests that people who are less aware of their illness tend to perceive less need for treatment (Cuffel, Alford, Fischer and Owen, 1996), to have longer episodes of medication non-adherence, to suffer more severe symptoms, and to experience more frequent hospitalizations (Olfson, Marcus, Wilk, and West, 2006). In addition, unawareness of illness may also adversely affect one's ability to benefit from rehabilitation as well as one's ability to function and relate to others (Francis and Penn, 2001; Lysaker, Bryson and Bell, 2002).

Many explain unawareness of illness in terms of a neurally-based inability to employ abstract concepts and/or a natural wish to ward off the social stigma linked to schizophrenia (Lysaker, Lancaster, Davis and Clements, 2003). Regardless of its etiology, lack of insight seems to intensify dialogical compromises of the kind we've been discussing, and in two ways. Imagine having a vague sense that one was faring less well than before, but maintaining the belief that the likely symptom of and thus key to one's diminishment was irrelevant to one's situation. Presuming one's assessment was mistaken, one would continue to fare poorly, and perhaps waste time addressing unrelated situations. This is precisely the kind of scenario we think occurs when people lack insight into, or an awareness of the symptoms associated with schizo-phrenia – the dialogical compromises they affect continue unabated. The point is not simply that such folk are unlikely to seek help, but also that their lack of awareness prevents the development of a meta-position, for example, self-as-ill, which could help them interpret and thus delimit the influence of the unusual experiences and/or beliefs they find themselves having.

Lack of insight into one's condition is also likely to intensify social alienation. Without a plausible account of one's trouble, it would be nearly impossible to talk to others about one's experiences and the difficulties that often surround them. Imagine Grieg describing his divorce without acknowledging the impact that his hallucinations and refusal to seek treatment may have had upon his wife. Imagine Webern telling a neighbor who had known him for many years that despite everything that had happened to him, he was 'fine'. In these cases, we don't see how any significant and enlivening dialogue could take place about events clearly central to the lives of both men. The addressees would probably respond with either explicit incredulity or a polite attempt to redirect or even exit the conversation. If so, then insofar as Grieg or Webern's symptoms were manifest in their relations with others, an inability to recognize them as such should lead to varying degrees of social alienation, and for both parties. As we've argued, social alienation deprives one of the interanimating presence of others as well intersubjective recognition, both of which are integral to the flow of character-positions and meta-positions. If one's neighbors avoid one, it is difficult to be, or regard oneself as a neighbor. This means, then, that due to the social alienation it affects, lack of insight into or awareness of illness is likely to negatively impact the interanimating flow of self-positions among those suffering from schizophrenia.

Mutual impact of insight and dialogical compromise

Like positive and negative symptoms, it strikes us that lack of awareness of or insight into illness can be exacerbated by dialogical compromises. For Grieg to regard his delusion as a delusion, he must be capable of generating the meta-position, self-as-ill, which would seem to require a distinct self-position not swept up in the symptoms of his illness. In other words, he has to both perceive his delusional thought and take the stance of someone who can not only dispute it, but also treat it as a symptom. With diminished dialogical capacities, and especially within a monological self-organization, the task of self-awareness should prove especially difficult. If one's character and meta-positions fade away, perhaps because they are colonized by one particular position, e.g. self-as-persecuted, and/or devolve into a cacophonous whirl, then one loses the kind of relative distance from one's condition, which insight into it as illness requires.

Dialogical compromises might also establish a situation wherein lack of insight could serve as a coping strategy. If dialogical breakdowns lead to a sense of self as diminished, and particularly with regard to one's agency, awareness of illness could be overwhelming. Recall that one of our central claims is that sense of self derives from the interanimating play of self-positions. As that play proves increasingly disordered, sense of self will suffer, finding little to hold onto besides its diminishment. As we saw with Frank, the thought that one is nothing but diminishment can be devastating. So, it may be that a refusal to see one's symptoms as symptoms allows one a sense of self that is disoriented and diminished, but at least not the nothingness that seemed to loom on the edges of Frank's paranoia. (In this regard, lack of insight, like positive and negative symptoms, may be more than a simple deficit in self-organizations aligned with schizophrenia).

Summary

At the outset of this chapter, we asked whether a dialogical account of schizophrenia could help us understand the emergence of symptoms, or whether, while preserving schizophrenia's first-person dimensions, it led to another dualistic dead end. In reply, we have suggested that several characteristic symptoms (complex verbal hallucinations, systematized delusions, blunted affect, lack of volition, and poor insight) might exacerbate and be exacerbated by dialogical compromises. Our claim then is that while symptoms and self-experience may be distinct in schizophrenia, they may also mutually affect one another via the thread of dialogical disturbance. Symptoms may disrupt dialogue, which disrupts self-experience, and/or a disruption in dialogue may both compromise sense of self and exacerbate symptoms, all leading to potentially grave psychosocial trajectories. If this is the case, then addressing schizophrenia with resources provided by dialogical theory enables us to see how one's experiences of the illness are part and parcel of its course and development, even if one believes, as we do, that neurological processes are also integral to the onset and course of the disease.

Endnotes

1 A sticky, epistemological question arises once we realize that a thought could be delusional and true. This isn't the context for an in-depth consideration of the matter, but whether a thought is delusional seems to turn in part on the quality of one's justifications for entertaining it. If so, delusions would involve thoughts that strike one's community as wildly implausible, and for which no compelling evidence can be provided. This refinement is important, for otherwise we'll find ourselves terming scientific revolutionaries like Galileo delusional.

2 We should note that Webern probably also experiences complex verbal hallucinations and delusions which are mildly systematized. In his case, then, we may be able to see interactions between positive and negative symptoms with particular impacts upon dialogue processes.

3 Of note, in this context 'insight' does not denote an awareness of unconscious motives or self-contradiction. It only refers to awareness of illness, i.e., the acceptance of the consensually validated understanding of the phenomena in question.

Chapter 6

Dialogical compromise and psychosocial dysfunction

In Chapter 5 we suggested that a dialogical conception of schizophrenia broadens our understanding of many of the disorder's landmark, objective features. We proposed, in particular, that a vicious cycle of mutual exacerbation exists between (a) dialogical compromises and experiences of self-diminishment and (b) a range of positive and negative symptoms. If we are right, and if, as we also propose, the two sets of phenomena are irreducible to one another, then a thorough understanding of vulnerability to one requires an understanding of vulnerability to the other. Moreover, it evidences that dialogical theory not only enables us to appreciate the first-person dimensions of schizophrenia, but it also begins to show us how those dimensions are part and parcel of the illness.

In this chapter, we'll explore whether dialogical compromises and experiences of self-diminishment have any bearing on a second set of objective disturbances, namely, psychosocial dysfunction, a matter of great concern to people with schizophrenia and to their families. As noted in Chapter 1, difficulties functioning socially and/or vocationally are a defining feature of schizophrenia. Such difficulties include problems establishing and maintaining friendships or romantic attachments as well as persisting at work. With the development of the illness, as illustrated in some of the case histories presented earlier, contacts with others may vanish. In fact, inactivity may become a way of life. Regardless, the psychosocial difficulties involved in schizophrenia are enduring, pervasive, and may involve impoverished relationships with family, friends, and acquaintances across any number of settings including the home, community, school, and work.

The psychosocial deficits found in schizophrenia form an enormously complex phenomenon with multiple social and biological roots, many of which seem quite distant from people's sense of self. For instance, social dysfunction may likely reflect, in part, general difficulties that many disabled people face. With schizophrenia, as with any other major medical condition, many afflicted people find themselves shunned by the world. Support from others is often lacking, and at times they feel avoided and rejected, if not cast aside and treated as if they were 'unclean' or carried an active contagion. Without supportive relationships, therefore, functional capacity may wane in schizophrenia, as it does for people with chronic pain, breast cancer, or AIDS. As their relationships dwindle, disabled people, including those with schizophrenia, may feel increasingly isolated, and conclude that, despite the best of their abilities, they are doomed to marginalization at work and in their communities.

A number of other qualities specifically linked to schizophrenia may also complicate workplace activities and relations with others. With reduced cognitive flexibility and idiosyncratic ways of making sense of the world, social situations that were previously comfortable and easily negotiable may prove frightening and be experienced as opportunities for embarrassment and rejection (Lysaker and Hammersly, 2006). Due to cognitive deficits, people with schizophrenia may also find it difficult to decode social interactions, to judge the feelings and intentions of others, and to intuit what they should say or do in specific situations (e.g., Bryson, Bell and Lysaker, 1997; Carter and Flesher, 1995; Grieg, Bryson and Bell, 2004; Penn et al., 1997). A joke offered by a co-worker, in what is commonly seen as a playful situation, may feel like a personal insult. In a tense situation, a vaguely threatening comment may be indistinguishable from a friendly overture. Or the social rules that define when a joke is appropriate, or when and how one should express love or disgust, may seem ungraspable. Thus, psychosocial function may be compromised not only by the onslaught of discriminatory social forces but also as result of measurable cognitive deficits that reduce one's chances of understanding complex social interactions.

Given the enormity of the issue of psychosocial dysfunction among people with schizophrenia and among disabled people in general, we will not offer a comprehensive theory of social dysfunction, just as the last chapter did not pursue a complete account of positive and negative symptoms. Instead, we'll explore whether a dialogical account of schizophrenia can supplement and broaden existing knowledge about psychosocial dysfunction and help us understand its persistence. To be clear, we acknowledge the effects of stigma as well as the debilitating power of anxious confusions that accompany overwhelming social situations. We will suggest, however, that dialogical compromises and experiences of diminishment lead people to experience intimacy and closeness with others in a manner that leaves them even more vulnerable to alienation and dysfunction.

In venturing our hypothesis, we will specifically consider whether the types of self-disruption that we regard as broadly characteristic of schizophrenia could intensify a person's vulnerability to stigma. We will then ask whether, at the level of intimate interaction, diminished dialogical capacities affect how people experience knowing and being known by another. Do the kinds of compromises we have discussed limit one's abilities to undergo what is entailed when we encounter a friend, colleague, or lover, and what is entailed when we encounter another who knows us? Finally, are dialogical compromises meaningfully bound to the issue of persistence at life tasks? In each case, we will answer in the affirmative, which suggests that psychosocial dysfunction marks a second site where the first-person dimensions of schizophrenia robustly interact with the illness's objective dimensions.

Stigma, oppressive power relationships, and dialogical compromise

As noted, stigma (Markowitz, 1998; Wright *et al.*, 2000) and oppressive power relationships (Rudge and Morse, 2001) have been widely identified as powerful antecedents of poor social and vocational functioning in schizophrenia. Stigma refers to stereotyped beliefs about people with mental illness, which include views that mental illness is synonymous with dangerousness, unpredictability, and incompetence. To assume that a mentally ill person cannot manage his or her own funds, or that he or she should be spoken to like a child, is to perpetuate stigma. Stigma, which can be found across all levels of social division, is more than an inaccurate group of beliefs. Stigma leads people who do not suffer from psychoses to avoid those who do. Moreover, it demoralizes those people with schizophrenia who come to accept these stereotypes as true (Lysaker, Roe and Yanos, 2007).

The term 'oppressive power relationships' names a related phenomenon. It refers to institutionally specified interactions in which people with severe mental illness feel controlled by the form or type of interaction occurring. For instance, while meeting with a case manager or interacting with a police officer, some people may feel as if they are being defined as mentally ill and consequently spoken to or treated in a manner that suggests they are less valuable members of society. They may have been offered unsolicited advice, or the manager/officer may have assumed the right to direct them. In either case, the institutionally affiliated person is acting in a way that exceeds the bounds within which people generally act to control or influence others, which denigrates the recipient of the behavior.

Stigma and oppressive power relationships prevent people with schizophrenia from relating to others as equals, and they create tangible barriers to meeting basic needs. If others view one as dangerous or unpredictable because of one's mental illness, and if they take one's illness to define most of who one is (to the point of regarding one as a 'what'), then they are more likely to avoid one. In particular, they are unlikely to hire one or see one's side of things if one gets into legal, financial, or medical trouble. Consequently, one will have less access to the networks of support that are integral to a stable, meaningful life.

With this conception of stigma in mind, our question is: would the effects of stigma prove more destructive if one were already undergoing dialogical disruptions and experiencing oneself as diminished? Inversely, could stigma contribute to a sense of oneself as diminished? We think so, and in both cases. There is empirical evidence that experiences of stigmatization correlate with decrements in self-esteem and a sense of being less than others (Dickerson *et al.*, 2002; Markowitz, 1998; Wright *et al.*, 2000). It also seems likely that people with limited dialogical capacity might be especially vulnerable to the effects of stigma. If people have fewer dialogical resources, they might find it more difficult to refute a discourse (i.e., to say 'that's not me', or 'I'm more than that'), if it carries the weight of expert medical advice and society at large, and if, at the outset, it disqualifies the 'mad' from rational deliberation, perhaps even interpreting their objections to stigmatizing behavior and unjust institutional treatment as further manifestations of illness.

Let us elaborate and further specify our suggestion. If one already regards oneself as diminished, i.e., holds a meta-position like 'self-as-less-than-before', then stigma, which presents one as less than others, would seem to confirm that self-regard. One used to be like others, but with the onset of mental illness, one no longer is. Moreover, stigma might offer some odd solace insofar as the identification 'mentally ill' purports to explain one's diminishment, thereby bringing an aura of order to the disordered play of self-positions. At the level of sense of self, therefore, those with schizophrenia seem primed for stigmatization.

It also seems that stigma is well groomed to intensify experiences of diminishment. In order to live with and recover from a prolonged mental illness, one usually must accept that one is limited by 'the boundaries that mental illness has placed upon life and … that most of the experiences that define essential humankind are still attainable' (Corrigan 2003, p. 349). Thus, in moving towards wellness, one will need a meta-positional sense of self-as-ill and as-more-than-ill, the latter enabling one to weave together whatever non-ill self-facets are provided through one's various character-positions, for example, self-as-mechanic, gardener, beloved-sister, etc. Stigmatization seems to block such moments of positive regard, however (Roe, 2001). Analogously to how positive symptoms might colonize a self who is suffering from compromised dialogical processes, pushing them in the direction of a monological self-organization, stigma could colonize a dialogically compromised self at the meta-positional level, reinforcing self-facets that are in line with stigma, for example, self-as-incompetent, and undermining those that are not, thereby weakening one's resistances to dialogical compromises. In other words, by trumping potentially affirmative self-disclosures, stigma may disincline one to synthesize the competency one shows in various character-positions into a meta-position that might rival one's stigmatized identity. In fact, it might disincline one to narrate one's life story altogether. After all, what is there to find if one is thoroughly mentally ill? If this is true, if stigmatization undermines the generation of meta-positions in general, it will further corrode one's reflectively pursued intrapersonal dialogues, even as such corrosions leave one all the more vulnerable to stigma.

If we turn to other dialogical processes, we find a similar cycle of vulnerability and intensification. Schizophrenia often leads to a sense of self as diminished because a disrupted flow of self-positions fails to provide one with even those pre-reflectively operative senses of self that are aligned with character-positions. In a cacophonous self-organization, disorder is the rule, and it trumps whatever sense of self one might receive from social roles, thus leaving one vulnerable to stigma. In a barren self-organization, the monotone of barely animate persistence rules the day, thus robbing one of a wide range of self-disclosures able to evidence that one is more than what one's stigmatized identity conveys. Finally, monological self-organizations carry every self-relation into their totalizing narratives. This may provide a point of resistance to stigmatization, but only through the very meta-position that everyone else regards as symptomatic of one's illness. Thus, even at the level of character-positions and their pre-reflectively operative interanimating play, stigma might find little to contest its negative self-conceptions if dialogical processes are compromised. Inversely, and this just repeats the point from above, stigmatization contributes a socially sanctioned 'you are nothing more than this' to the disorienting experiences that accompany breakdowns in dialogical processes. Through its objectifying, totalizing equation of one with one's illness, it thus trumps, in whatever reflective moments arise, experiences that suggest that one is more than 'mad'.

In this context, let us return to Glass, whose self-organization conformed to the barren model. A consideration of his self-presentations suggests that his sense of self reflects the influence of oppressive power relationships. Early in his psychotherapy, he asserted that he was empty, and reported that doctors had told him that he was ill and could not work. To anyone who doubted this, he offered the challenge, 'Just look at my chart,' which suggests that his chart had more to say about who he was than he did. In such conversations, he also indicated that he generally had not been included in discussions about his illness. He also spoke of how, on an inpatient ward some six months earlier, he had been watching everyone else come and go. He had no idea why he remained where he was, and it never dawned on him that he had the right to inquire about whether he too might move. Similarly, he reported having given his assent the last time a psychiatrist had recommended a change in his medication, but only because he feared that he might lose certain benefits if he asserted himself.

Glass was quite explicit: he was mentally ill, and there was nothing else to know about him. He did not believe that any meaningful future lay ahead of him, and he had little to say to himself or others. With regard to what he had to say and do, he felt that it followed from instructions he had been given. When pressed to explain what it meant that he was 'mentally ill and that is all', he seemed surprised and dismissed the question as meaningless. On our view, this indicates not only a lack of rival self-positions, but also the fact that others had never sought his opinion about this matter. Instead they engaged him as a patient to be treated. If so, by not soliciting self-positions that ran against his sense of self, Glass's caretakers inadvertently reinforced his belief that 'self-as-ill' was all he was, and this helped suspend him in a barely differentiated cloudbank of minimal self-positions and blunted affect, which only further evidenced his diminishment.

Of course, someone with schizophrenia could withdraw from any stigmatizing interaction, including those that employ the illness label. If so, if Glass had avoided relationships mediated by stigmatizing beliefs, he might have had more to say about what he thought and felt; he might also have had greater hope for the future. However, if he privileged self-positions linked with his abilities, this would risk a different kind of isolation, the kind faced by those who lack insight into their illness. Without any acknowledgement of illness, it would be impossible to discuss and address his struggles with an eye on their roots, which could easily lead to great social dysfunction. If this produced intense isolation, stigmatization might still prevail as he, since others were unable to engage him on his own terms, struggled to interpret his lack of meaningful attachments.

One sees something quite close to this last trajectory in Grieg's self-presentations, which oscillate between self-as-entirely-ill and not-ill-at-all. As noted, Grieg alternately acknowledged, without any awareness of contradiction, that he was (a) alone, distressed, and incapable of action, and (b) that there was nothing wrong with him. In the same session, he would commonly present himself as utterly disabled, and then, a bit later, as doing quite well. He would begin: 'I can do nothing ... too much medication ... it's the shock treatments ... I need more shock treatments' and a few minutes later, he would say '... but everyone likes me ... there's nothing I can't do. I stop by the school and see if they need a soccer coach—I was a good player—or I could go back to church and go on a mission.' Despite their contradictory nature, each response effects the same relation to illness. There is nothing to be said or done about it, which means that, demeaning treatment at the hands of others (which, over time, contributes to a sense of oneself as diminished), either bewilders Grieg, or he simply accepts it as a just recognition of who he has become. In either case, he remains vulnerable to stigma and unjust treatment within the power relationships to which he is continually subjected.

In summary, then, our claim is that one encumbered with dialogical compromises and a sense that one has diminished is likely to be more vulnerable to stigma and oppressive power relations as well as to their disabling effects. It is also likely that those effects intensify dialogical compromises and the sense of being diminished. If so, and this is a more general point, it would appear that social injustice and the first-person dimensions of schizophrenia mutually influence each other over the course of the illness.

Knowing the other and dialogical compromise

As discussed, it is difficult for people with schizophrenia to know the other, to fathom his or her intentions, emotions, and/or thoughts. Moreover, social interactions can be bewildering for people with schizophrenia, to the point that a brief engagement can prove overwhelming. In either case, experiences like these lead people to avoid social interactions, a fate that, as noted, deprives them of needed support and services. Moreover, it produces feelings of intense loneliness and isolation.

Certainly, difficulties in interpreting others may stem in part from the compromises in neurocognitive function that characterize schizophrenia. With reduced capacities to determine what is relevant from irrelevant, to call to mind the complexities of context, and to think flexibly about the person in question, it would be difficult to make sense of even moderately complicated social situations. Yet this may not be the whole story. Knowing another does not involve one disembodied essence accepting facts or a transmission about another disembodied essence (Stanghellini, 2004). We are not computers sharing information. As suggested by simulation theory (Gallese, 2001), knowing something about someone else involves complex cortical processes reliant upon mirror neurons that appear to simulate what another might be feeling or thinking, though not by representing those phenomena. Rather, mirror neurons appear to give us the analogous thoughts and feelings, thus enabling us to undergo what the other is undergoing, e.g., we feel embarrassed along with their embarrassment, or know their loneliness by feeling a bit lonely ourselves.

Knowing another involves other interactions as well. As suggested in Chapter 3, the people we encounter animate various self-positions, and in various ways. At work, depending upon whom one is talking to and what that person says, one can be drawn into self-as-worker, self-as-mentor, self-as-concerned-citizen, or self-as-envious. In order to address a colleague's work, we'll have to address them through our overlapping roles, and with various meta-positions in play, e.g., self-as-charitable. Of course, attempting to know someone is a two-way street. Our colleague's response may animate self-as-administrator and/or and self-as-competitive. Self-positions also can be animated in more unpredictable ways. Our colleague may look like an old, disloyal friend and animate self-as-betrayed. In short, seeking out others puts our self-positions constantly on the move, and in ways that are often unintended and nearly impossible to anticipate.

Given the movement among self-positions that engaging others requires, even at a casual level, it seems likely that someone who finds it difficult to move among self-positions in a coherent manner (that is, someone for whom ongoing intrapersonal dialogue is a struggle) may find the experience of engaging another confusing. Beyond wondering what others mean or what the situation dictates, encountering others may be dizzying and even threatening if their presence elicits aspects of oneself, which then have to participate in an already tenuous and wavering interanimating play. Our suggestion, then, is that efforts to engage others may evoke self-positions that people with schizophrenia have difficulty integrating into existing plays among other self-positions. For instance, even the blandest, most innocuous support group meeting might require one to move between self-as-mentally-ill, self-as-roommate, and self-as-peacemaker. Simultaneously, still other self-positions might be evoked without being integral to one's plans (e.g., self-as-lonely, self-as-misunderstood). If one then fails to negotiate the switches that must occur if one is to successfully address others, confusion could easily arise and imperil whatever intra- and interpersonal dialogues had been operative. If it were already hard to keep intrapersonal dialogue alive and to ward off cacophony, barrenness or monologue, addressing someone who animated meta-positions like 'self-as-jealous' or organism-positions like 'self-as-aroused' might prove too much to handle, and irrespective of whether those were predictable occurrences. And in the ensuing disorder, a feeling of even greater dissolution or diminishment might result if one were unable to find a stable position from which to assess the emerging blooming, biting confusion. In short, attempting to know others may undermine compromised dialogical processes, and the resulting confusion and alienation may further destabilize already compromised dialogical processes and deepen experiences of diminishment.

Early in his psychotherapy, Purcell suggested that interaction with others was overwhelming; it evoked more than he could handle. He explained:

> I'm just a speck ... a speck on somebody's friendship or something. It's too late to change a lifestyle into a system or more... I mean to be with an individual and never leave the ground, a complete human being. I mean you get messed up over interacting with others, seems like it swings both ways.... you've got nothing to contribute and it's not worth another person's time.

And then months later:

> Not all the time do you get a good picture of what you want to say. You speak one thing and say something else. Good is bothered by my bad alone. It is like trading places or trying to settle yourself, trying to become settled so you make roots or have a foundation … something that is either common or that I can work at something … too many things about someone's faith … moving in time and being stationary, see what I mean … transporting… for me to put up with myself and to come to grips it might be pushing a lot of things out of the way.

In Purcell's self-presentation, we hear (a) intersubjectively generated confusion and anxiety due to weak dialogical organizations, and (b) weakening dialogical processes as a result of intersubjectively generated confusion. When he addressed others, Purcell was unable to find any footing, and so, whatever comfort might come from being around them was negated by the anxiety their presence provoked. But the problem isn't just that he believed that he had nothing to offer. In the presence of others, he found it difficult to know what he wanted to say, and found himself 'trading places' and 'transporting', but not in a way that amounted to a 'system', as he says in the initial remarks. Rather, what began as one thing became something else, that is, the flow of conversation became too difficult to follow, and he lost something that could be in 'common', that he could 'work at'. It is thus unsurprising (if heart rending) to find him later confess to being unsettled, and to the point that he cannot 'put up with himself', which we interpret to mean that in such exchanges, his self-disclosure is too painful to bear. In fact, to our ears, Purcell's unsettled condition suggests the beginnings of a cacophonous self-organization, one no doubt already looming, but clearly intensified by his efforts to engage others.

Looking more generally at the psychosocial dimensions of schizophrenia, it now seems that dialogical compromise not only enters into a reciprocal relation with stigmatization, but with another mode of social dysfunction, namely, profound anxiety and confusion while engaging others. Like stigmatization, whether informal or bound to oppressive power relationships, the dialogical disruptions that such engagements further may intensify psychosocial dysfunction more generally, the inference being that compromises in the dialogical self will likely lead people to refrain from trying to meet and know others given the degree of fright and anxiety those efforts produce.

Being known by the other and dialogical compromise

Purcell's comments disclose a further and equally important issue. Being known also may prove disorienting and destabilizing. Not that knowing and being known are discrete events. Except in unusual circumstances – for example, spying or voyeurism – it is difficult to imagine one process commencing without the other. We offer the distinction in order to throw into starker relief some of the challenges that intersubjectivity poses for those who suffer from schizophrenia. Not only do people with schizophrenia have difficulty seeking out and sustaining attachments, but also, even the approach of others can be a source of unease and pain. In this section, then, we'll return to the issue of intersubjectivity, focusing on scenarios when the other, intentionally or inadvertently, initiates the engagement.

As we argued in Chapter 3, just as coming to know others animates self-positions, others evoke aspects of self as they behold us. Moreover, social life not only solicits self-positions, it also foists them upon us, and we have to confront and deal with the many self-positions evoked and/or created in how others engage us. From a dialogical point of view, the address of the other must be taken up within the intrapersonal conversations that in part constitute character. After interpolating the address of another, one must accept, modify, or reject it with whatever resources one's self-positions provide. Suppose a disheveled man approaches you on the way to work. He explains that he's run out of gas and needs $20 to get back on the road. In such an instance, you probably receive his address via a character-position like self-as-worker because you're on the way to work and because the request concerns money, but insofar as the address calls for a response, it probably also animates some meta-positions, say self-as-progressive or self-as-charitable. Now, suppose that self-as-worker wins out. You're late, and your boss has been in a bad mood. You might initially feel bad, but not for long since you've witnessed this scam before.

Let's vary the scene. What if, as you pass, the man calls out, angrily: 'Can't you spare a few bucks for a fellow human being? God, I hate rich people!' Again, you keep walking, and as you do so, you chuckle at the thought of being regarded as rich. However, the attribution, self-as-fellow-human-being rattles around your head all day. In this instance, the address of another more or less inserts two potential meta-positions into your self-organization. One you dismiss rather easily. But you struggle with self-as-fellow-human-being, a bit lost in its vagueness and implications. We note this scenario because it evidences that the address of another not only can animate existing self-positions, but can also interject more or less new ones. It also shows how pre-existent self-positions can be animated by these inter-polations, and how pre-existent positions help orient our reception of and response to interpolated ones.[1]

Consider how one might respond to the panhandling scenario if one's dialogical resources were compromised, particularly along the lines we've associated with schizophrenia. As in the case of trying to know another, any animation of self-positions might prove disorient-ing for one with a more or less cacophonous self-organization and lead to socially dysfunctional responses, for example, replying to the request for money with remarks about one's employment history (sparked by the animation of self-as-worker) or family troubles (sparked by the animation of self-as-neglected). In the case of a monological self-organization, one will have a limited repertoire of responses, and thus again reply in a manner that seems socially dysfunctional, perhaps replying to the request for money with an accusation of persecution, or with the remark: 'Yes, I could tell you recognized me. We may have known each other in a previous life.' Moreover, the address of others will animate self-facets beyond the reach of one's monologue, which may threaten its coherence, as will the refusal of others to recognize the legitimacy of one's monological narrative and the responses they fund. Because barren self-organizations involve a minimal range of self-positions, and in their most minimal form, one wouldn't expect such people to struggle as much with the ways in which social life animates self-positions. Nevertheless, one would expect someone with a barren self-organization to have a general sense of not being able to keep up with all the action, much like Webern found himself while watching the basketball game. It was not a source of great anxiety, but he had trouble tracking what transpired around him.

What about when the address of another interpolates into one's self-organization a more or less novel self-position? Without an array of self-positions that might contextualize and resist the interpolation, one might come to feel colonized by the other's address, which is something that many people suffering from schizophrenia attest to feeling (Pao-Nie, 1979; Parnas and Handset, 2003). If so, the result would mirror the kind of scenario that Sartre (1956) made famous in his discussions of the gaze of the other. One loses one's sense of self to whatever position the other's gaze (or address) introduces into one's self-organization, which might affect something like a temporary monological self-organization wherein other self-facets wither in the face of the interpolated position. Except, in this instance, the alien nature of the self-position would be part and parcel of its presence, which might prompt the emergence of an organism-position centered by intense anxiety. Even if it did not, it remains likely that such an experience would contribute to the more general experience of diminishment.

Purcell seems to exemplify this phenomenon. If we return to his claim, 'I am just a speck ... a speck on somebody's friendship or something,' and contextualize it in terms of other remarks, we find that initially this is not a self-attribution. Rather, he believes that others regard him as a speck and so he regards himself as a speck. What others see him to be is what he sees himself to be. He elaborates:

> If you use yourself raw and they always got an impression of you, or they see your expression or loss of content ... it's very frustrating because if it's too late in life to get them, you feel down ... it's hard to put yourself on the incline.

Two things strike us here. First, the regard of others seems to be a source of friction for Purcell, one that leaves him 'raw' and again without footing on a slope (or 'incline'), which suggest anxiety and frustration. Second, note the immediate shift from 'they always got an impression of you' to 'they see your ... loss of content'. This is precisely the phenomenon under discussion. Others regard us and we disappear in that regard, but not to the point that we can't experience ourselves as having disappeared, hence Purcell's feeling of being worn down, even away.

In this context, we'd also like to direct your attention to the case of Wagner, which we have discussed in a previous article (Lysaker, Johannesen, and Lysaker, 2005). Although he lives a more or less stable life, he has experienced positive and cognitive symptoms since his mid-20s, which have contributed to a cacophonous self-organization. In several pronounced ways, Wagner has reported being overwhelmed by self-positions from very definite contexts, namely church (self-as-sinful) and the hospital (self-as-schizophrenic). Remarkably, he has also expressed concerns that contact with drug addicts would make him a drug addict. Not that he would start taking drugs, but that their identity would replace his. In other words, just entertaining the thought of such a life/persona was sufficient to threaten whatever sense of self he was able to maintain.

Because monological self-organizations are ruled by totalizing narratives, colonizing interpolations shouldn't arise in such instances. Instead, others that address one will be cast as either ally or enemy, and within a univocal context. While this should affect social function, it won't in the way that we are now considering. One also wouldn't expect colonizing interpolations in barren self-organizations. In these cases, no self-position has a particularly dominant role, and thus no interpolation should prove overwhelming. Of course, recurring flat affect can lead to psychosocial dysfunction, but once again, not in the way we are now considering. It would seem then that only those whose dialogical compromises have a cacophonous character are particularly vulnerable to experience colonizing interpolations.

Considered generally, being addressed by others appears to initiate the same kind of cycles that we found in the cases of stigma and attempts to know others. The diminished dialogical capacity that characterizes schizophrenia undermines one's ability to successfully respond to the varied and dynamic intersubjective tasks that run through social life. Whether in explicit or implicit exchanges, self-positions are animated and interpolated, which requires one to keep pace with an evolving and often conflicted sense of self, but this is precisely what those suffering from schizophrenia often cannot do. It is unsurprising, therefore, that engagements with others are often a source of anxiety, despair, avoidance reactions, and even feelings of dissolution among people with schizophrenia, phenomena that only intensify experiences of diminishment, often to profound degrees. As Wagner put the matter, rather drily: 'I have a problem with identity.' Moreover, anxiety, avoidance, experiences of colonization and the like seem to contribute to a downward spiral of dialogical disarray, which feeds back into psychosocial dysfunction. As his anxiety mounts, Purcell's cacophony intensifies, which only feeds his psychosocial dysfunction, leaving him all the more disconsolate about who he has and continues to become.

Commitment and persistence amid dialogical compromise

Let us now consider a different order of psychosocial dysfunction, namely, committing to and persisting in action. In the context of schizophrenia, these difficulties do not just refer to the process of obtaining jobs or even considering appropriate life goals. Instead, they concern problems committing to and persisting at a task or extended course of action once it has begun. Our question then, is: can dialogical disturbances also undermine one's ability to follow through with tasks given the predictable ups and downs that characterize most extended activities, whether they are matters of work, exercise, or leisure?

In order to explore this phenomenon, let's consider Glass, Grieg, and Purcell. Each has a unique clinical portrait and distinct self-organization, namely, barren, monological, and cacophonous. Yet each reports a strikingly similar, manifold inability to follow through with a course of action. Regardless of whether Grieg presents himself as sick or well, he makes little progress towards returning to work or persisting in projects that he identifies as important, such as following through with a recommended diet and exercise regimen. Glass and Purcell seem even less able to commit to courses of action. Both state that they want to work, but neither ever applies for a job. On their own account, putting in an application is not in any way undesirable. Nor does either seem particularly guilty of procrastination, or riddled by a nagging or obsessive doubt. Moreover, in the abstract, each recognizes that humans can and should commit to action. However, despite the suffering that results from their inaction, they cannot commit to extended courses of action and, in clinical settings, if they ever hint at some inclination to commit, it is reversed moments later.

Remarkably, each man describes the process of commitment to and persistence in action in similar terms. It is profoundly threatening. In fact, each seems to consider himself insufficient to survive action, that is, the prospects of extended action – taking a job, entering into a relationship, or regularly pursuing a hobby, reinforces a sense of self as diminished, as no longer capable of such things. Purcell and Glass both hint strongly that commitment to an action will overwhelm them. Purcell again speaks of being rubbed raw, and Glass, ever in a cloudbank, speaks of having 'commitment terror', and intimates that if he were to emerge from the inactivity of the cloudbank he could be destroyed.

In our view, the dialogical compromises that we regard as integral to schizophrenia may render commitment and persistence more or less unimaginable for those with the disorder. First, insofar as extended actions involve recurring and novel social engagements, the same issues that arise in intersubjective exchanges will arise here. In other words, if one is disinclined to engage or be engaged by others, one very likely will be disinclined to do things like seek out jobs. However, the sense that intersubjective life is threatening is not the only or even principal snag here. Rather, there is something about committing to and persisting in extended action itself that looms menacingly when schizophrenia is present.

First, commitment to action requires some minimal order among self-positions such that the needs of the character and meta-positions associated with the task in question are given priority over other desires, inclinations, and responses. Interestingly, monological self-organizations do not seem to derail initial commitments to action. Grieg is very able to plan and initiate futures. So too is Scarlatti, whom we've discussed elsewhere (Lysaker, Buck and Ringer, 2007), and who also has a monological self-organization. He often assembles elaborate plans. For example, he once decided to open a sports memorabilia shop, and went to the lengths of acquiring thousands of baseball cards that he intended to sell. It would seem, then, that monological self-organizations provide a strong enough sense of self to initiate courses of extended action (though persistence is another matter).

In a cacophonous self-organization, commitment to extended actions is significantly more difficult. Because stability and order among self-positions is fleeting for people subjected to cacophony, commitment to action can be tenuous, the future as jumbled as the present. Purcell occasionally pursued things on his own initiative, for example, attending psychotherapy sessions and enrolling in a vocational rehabilitation program, but beyond that, he had profound difficulty initiating the kind of extended actions one associates with adult life. As noted, the very thought terrified him. He presented himself as having been 'scared into a cage', and he regarded whatever futures he might initiate as very risky and profoundly destabilizing. 'I mean for me to put up with myself and to come to grips, it might be pushing a lot of things out of the way.' When asked about his wish to have a more stable life, he replied, continuing the previous line of thought: 'If I get rid of one thing and I make room for another thing, I am not grateful to be. I don't know how my body is functioning against itself.' The image of a body against itself is painfully acute in this context. With the play of self-positions in wild disarray, it is exceedingly difficult to imagine and commit to a definite future.

In a barren self-organization, a different problem arises. Self-positions are action orientations, and they provide us, alongside meta-positions, with a storyline from which to weave our plans. Upon graduating from college, we did not just want 'jobs', we wanted to be a psychologist and a philosophy professor, and so we set about taking the steps needed for those positions. Not that we really knew what the future held, but on the basis of a rich character-position, i.e., self-as-student (and even more specifically, self-as-psychology-major and self-as-philosophy-major), we could imagine taking the next step. Self-as-graduate-student was a step towards a possible profession. We were thus able to commit in part because our proposed futures were clear extensions of existing character-positions, complemented no doubt by meta-positions like self-as-intellectual and self-as-helpful, as well as the character-position self-as-son, the latter inclining us to pursue something that would win our parents' approval. In other words, rich dialogical processes helped us articulate and pursue a definite future.

If we recall Glass, we find a different scene. Glass is someone who wants to do something, even something as specific as 'get a job' or 'have a relationship', but he lacks a sufficiently determinate array of character and meta-positions from which to assay that future. Glass meets possible partners, but he never courts any. He says:

> I want a commitment but at the same time I'm going in the opposite direction … I have hope but don't visit or call. I don't know what love is … Don't know about very much except that I'm afraid. I can't make anything work.

Glass seems paralyzed by not really knowing how to proceed. His future is thus as much a cloudbank as his present. No doubt his blunted affect plays a role here as well. As we noted in Chapter 5, without animating force, character-positions contract, and one's motivation to change loses much of its push and pull. The more general point, though, is that if one has only a small range of character-positions, and if they are minimal versions at that, it will prove extremely difficult to articulate a future to which one might commit.

Now let's explore a second way in which dialogical compromises might undermine the pursuit of extended action, this time focusing upon persistence at a task. Projects like acquiring a job or a new skill animate self-facets and positions, just like encounters with others do. If you work in a retail shop, for example, you will encounter new customers, co-workers with fluctuating moods, new products, busy days, slow days, frustrations, store politics, lost keys, products you might like to buy, the need to work when you don't want to, large amounts of cash, inopportune hunger, complex and occasionally malfunctioning cash registers, friends and/or family wanting discounts, etc. Thus, even if we take intersubjective complexity out of the equation, extended actions animate play among self-positions and loom as sites of ongoing and multifaceted self-disclosures. If play among self-positions is a source of pain and/or anxiety, as it is for many people with schizophrenia, one might very well avoid or flee such contexts.

Here then is our claim. People with schizophrenia have difficulty persisting in extended actions because such tasks confront them with overwhelming dialogical demands. In a cacophonous self-organization the ongoing interanimation of self-positions should produce anxiety and prove disorienting. In relating to customers, co-workers, supervisors, and the like, and in evolving contexts that also animate organism- and meta-positions, maintaining a predictable ordering of self-positions is a key to success. One cannot fly off the handle every time one gets angry or take extended breaks every time an acquaintance stops by. Moreover, certain self-positions, for example, self-as-religious-crusader, just don't belong in most workplaces, but finding order in all this multiplicity is often too much for those caught in a cacophonous whirl. In fact, Purcell never even got this far. He never actually applied for a job. Instead, his struggles with persistence arose within an attempt to establish an exercise regimen. Reflecting on himself and his efforts to do things, he said:

> If I put everything in perspective they would all be separate departments … If I can't make the transition, that won't give me time 'cause I won't understand … When I was young I used to feel that they knew everything even if I didn't. It's like stopping something you can't understand and trying to live a life as wanting to be capable.

Purcell wants to be capable of extended action, to be 'capable', but trying to be fractures him, leaving him confused. Under such conditions, it would be unsurprising if persisting at various tasks proved to be too difficult.

In a monological self-organization, the problem concerns too many disclosures that run counter to the content of the monologue. Grieg often moved between a delusionally elevated or denigrated self-regard, but on any given day, anyone will do well and poorly, which upsets what little order a monologue provides. Over time then, Grieg stopped working, and retreated to what he found to be stiller and calmer waters. Scarlatti, whom we mentioned a moment ago, and who acquired a great many baseball cards in order to open a shop, inevitably translated any interpersonal tension and dissonance into evidence of persecution. This not only undermines business relationships, it proves terribly taxing over time, which led Scarlatti to drop his ventures before they ever really get off the ground. Thus rather than opening the shop for sports memorabilia, his card collection is now in storage, and the prospect all but dead.

Summary

At the outset of this chapter, we asked whether compromises in dialogical capacities might play a role in psychosocial dysfunction. In reply, we suggested that social forces, which lead to dysfunction such as stigma and oppressive power relationships, may exacerbate and be exacerbated by dialogical compromises. We further argued that knowing and being known by another may animate more self-facets and positions than can be comfortably accommodated by one for whom intra- and interpersonal dialogue is a difficult task. As a result, intersubjectivity may be experienced as a threat and intimacy avoided, two effects that in turn seem to intensify dialogical breakdowns, which leads to a debilitating downward spiral that entrenches social dysfunction and deepens experiences of diminishment. Finally, when considering committed action within the community, we suggested that the dialogical demands of ongoing worldly interaction also bring disorder to the interanimating play of self-positions among people with schizophrenia, thereby leading them to avoid commitment and/or show a lack of perseverance over time. And while we didn't take the time to argue this, it seems evident that repeated failures of this sort not only contracts one's intra-and interpersonal dialogues, but also intensifies, with the help of stigma, experiences of diminishment.

Looking at the last two chapters as a whole, we have also argued that a dialogical approach to schizophrenia not only attends to and preserves the first-person dimensions of the illness, but also give us reason to suppose that these dimensions interact with third-person events over the course of the illness. In the cases of positive and negative symptoms, as well as psychosocial dysfunction, we have witnessed some of the ways in which self-disclosures, in the form of interanimating plays among self-positions, might render one vulnerable to and intensify the effects of oppressive social relationships, cognitive deficits, abnormal cortical activity, and so forth. These two chapters thus provide some more evidence for the claim that how one undergoes schizophrenia is relevant to how it unfolds over the course of one's life.

Endnotes

1 We should stress that the address need not be verbal in order to animate intrapersonal dialogue. If someone leers at us, or if another tries to stare us down in order to intimidate us (situations no doubt mediated by self-facets like gender, class, and race), structurally analogous processes should come into play. A leer may animate

a meta-position like self-as-sex-object, possibly even an organism-position, self-as-threatened, if the looker is particularly unpleasant and the context unsafe. It may also animate another meta-position, self-as-feminist, which, along with the organism-position, fuels justified anger. Regardless, we want to stress that others can address us without doing so verbally.

Chapter 7

Establishing and sustaining dialogue in individual psychotherapy

From the outset, our effort has been to respect the first-person dimensions of schizophrenia, focusing in particular on sense of self and the roles it might play in the course of illness. After reviewing various literatures, we argued in Chapter 3 that self-experience arises out of contextually situated intra-and interpersonal dialogues among three kinds of self-positions – character-positions, meta-positions, and organism-positions. On this view, sense of self is not given in an intuitive grasp of some stable, core self, but in a disclosure of some facet of the temporal, polyphonic constellation that each of us is. We then used this view to help explain why people who suffer from schizophrenia often experience themselves as diminished relative to their former selves.

In short, the illness, for manifold physiological and social reasons, compromises the dialogical processes wherein sense of self arises, leaving people feeling fragmented, broken, even destroyed. Keeping to our dialogical outlook, we also suggested that experiences of diminishment could arise in three different models of self-organization – barren, cacophonous, and monological – and that these models influence, in different ways, the development of positive and negative symptoms as well as psychosocial dysfunction. These latter observations also indicate a more general point. The first-person dimensions of schizophrenia are not simply subjective impressions of its objectivity: they contribute to the course of the illness, that is, how one undergoes schizophrenia is part and parcel of schizophrenia.

It would seem, then, that dialogical theory could contribute to how we conceptualize and diagnose schizophrenia. What, though, about the treatment of schizophrenia? If compromised dialogical capacities contribute to key facets of schizophrenia, how might one address those compromises?

In this chapter, we will present what we consider to be our theory's implications for psychotherapeutic treatments of schizophrenia. Specifically, we will consider how to help people both rekindle lost intra- and interpersonal dialogues and strengthen compromised dialogical capacities. We are focusing upon psychotherapy, because, by definition, it is a conversation between two or more people, and it often seeks the explicit goal of enriching a client's personal narratives (Fenton, 2000; Neimeyer and Raskin, 2000). It thus seems to have a dialogical core.

Because our focus is psychotherapy, it should be clear that our goal is not to introduce a radically new way of treating schizophrenia. Rather, we wish to explore whether our focus on dialogical compromises might enrich psychotherapy for schizophrenia. To that end, we begin by recalling psychotherapy's meteoric rise and decline as a treatment for schizophrenia. Next, we review some of the general problems that schizophrenia poses for those who would address it by way of psychotherapy. Third, we suggest that progress might be made if one widens psychotherapy for schizophrenia to include efforts to help people recover dialogical capacities.

The self and psychotherapy in schizophrenia
A brief history of psychotherapy for schizophrenia

As noted in Chapter 2, some psychoanalytic theories of schizophrenia propose that the psyche collapses into psychosis when it no longer can repress what were labeled 'primitive' or 'instinctual impulses'. Some also propose that schizophrenia is the direct result of faulty family dynamics or dysfunctional patterns of communication between parents and their children (for example, Mishler and Waxler, 1968). As detailed by Hartwell (1996), at a time when American society feared the growing independence of women, psychoanalytic theorists suggested that couples, composed of women who were consumed by their own needs and whose husbands were too weak to oppose them, lacked sufficient attunement to their children's needs, which rendered these children vulnerable to madness.

Alongside these assertions, some stressed that psychoanalytic psychotherapy was the treatment of choice for schizophrenia because psychoanalytic therapists possessed special knowledge regarding healthy human development. With this knowledge, they were the best guide for those seeking to recover from schizophrenia (Karon and van Denbos, 1981). Initially, recovering people might need to become intensely dependent upon their therapist, and they might even need to regress before they could develop properly (Rosen, 1947; Searles, 1965).

While not all psychodynamic thinkers agreed with these views, enough did that a firestorm ensued. Many professionals entirely rejected psychotherapy for schizophrenia on the grounds that it was oppressive, shamed families, promoted dysfunction and above all, derived from a groundless metapsychology (Drake and Sederer, 1986). Once touted as a panacea by psychoanalytic writers, psychotherapy for schizophrenia quickly fell off the academic radar. Once a treatment of choice, it is now rarely mentioned in the context of treatment for schizophrenia, and when it is, it is rarely presented as anything more than a vague supportive relationship intended to help people solve problems.

After the fall of psychoanalysis, psychotherapy for schizophrenia made something of a comeback with cognitive behavior therapy (CBT), which, since the 1980s, has gained some prominence (Beck *et al.*, 1979). CBT is a treatment which addresses psychological symptoms by assisting people to better recognize, correct and manage maladaptive patterns of thinking, feeling and behaving. It has found some success in the treatment of schizophrenia (Rector and Beck, 2002; Tarrier *et al.*, 2000; Tarrier and Wykes, 2004), where the emphasis on combating maladaptive beliefs seems to be beneficial (Davis and Lysaker, 2005). Also, a number of controlled trials have shown that CBT can reduce positive symptoms, negative symptoms, and length of hospital stay (Drury *et al.*, 1996; Sensky *et al.*, 2000).

Challenges for the psychotherapy for schizophrenia

Its tumultuous history aside, psychotherapy for schizophrenia also must confront some obvious hurdles. Individual psychotherapy, no matter how theoretically detailed or rule-governed, involves two people meeting to converse. Each arrives with his or her thoughts and feelings, and after a moment of silence, they talk. When the client has a specific problem, talking about it may be a relatively easy proposition. Before the onset of psychosis, Frank, whom we described in earlier chapters, initially came to therapy because he felt depressed and wanted to enjoy life again. Before his psychosis, he would arrive on time, sit, and discuss what depressed him. Like many other clients, he spoke about what gave him pleasure and what he thought he needed from other people. He talked about his struggles to love and forgive others and to manage his anxiety.

With the onset of psychosis, Frank's psychotherapy suddenly became profoundly more complex. Once he developed delusions of persecution, he no longer arrived, sat, and began talking. Instead, after sitting, he would look at the therapist belligerently. He would remain silent, hunched forward, or he would sit back and launch into a rage-filled diatribe about the forces persecuting him. As noted by many, and from multiple perspectives, a therapeutic alliance or working bond between the client and therapist is crucial to psychotherapy, and in the case of schizophrenia, that may be difficult to achieve (Fromm-Reichmann, 1954; Searles, 1965). People with schizophrenia may be unusually sensitive to any failure in empathic listening. The slightest inattentiveness, it has been suggested, can prove quite painful, leading the client to leave treatment or, as in the case of Frank, to withdraw from the therapist. More generally, a grave distrust may be harbored. This may mean that even the most well-intentioned gesture appears dangerous (Weiden and Havens, 1994). It may also mean that the idea of sharing personal material appears preposterous to the client.

The Boston Psychotherapy Study provides empirical evidence that confirms how difficult it is to pursue psychotherapy for schizophrenia (Gunderson *et al.*, 1984). The study involved over 150 participants with schizophrenia who were randomized to receive either psychoanalytic or supportive psychotherapy. Therapists were well-trained and supervised by a leader in the field of psychoanalytic psychotherapy for schizophrenia. Nevertheless, there was a stunning dropout rate. Over 40 percent did not complete the initial phase of treatment, and even more dropped out before the study's conclusion.

Alongside the thorny question concerning how to form relationships with clients who have schizophrenia, there is also the issue of what the client and therapist should discuss. Should they directly address the phenomenon of schizophrenia? After all, depressed clients can safely be presumed to address their depression. Yet such a presumption may be unwarranted in schizophrenia. First, the concept 'schizophrenia' lacks intuitive clarity, and even as a clinical term, it remains enormously complex and even slippery. Thus, while someone may know what it means to be anxious, the same cannot be said about being 'schizophrenic' – and the problem only intensifies if we recall that schizophrenia often makes it difficult to interpret the world in an orderly manner. Not only do cognitive deficits compromise conversation, but also, their presence may lead therapeutic dialogue to trigger rather than alleviate symptoms.

Neither Grieg, nor Glass, nor Purcell entered psychotherapy with an account of themselves as suffering from a biologically-based disorder with possible genetic roots that undermined their ability to cope with stress. None began by observing that they were failing to adequately distinguish their own thoughts from actual sensory experiences. Nor did any begin with a sense that they had anything like schizophrenia, and so they did not arrive seeking a treatment for a particular illness or even a clear set of symptoms. Rather, and this was well after their first visit, each revealed, in his own way, that he felt overwhelmed, stricken with anguish, and without any real sense for how to engage others. Eventually, each did decide that he had difficulties thinking about his own thinking, but this view only emerged after extended conversation about what he thought and felt, and how problematic it was to make sense of those thoughts and feelings. As one might suppose, then, the very phenomenon of schizophrenia makes addressing it in a psychotherapeutic setting extraordinarily difficult.

Dialogue when little dialogue is possible

Our entry into this history of controversies and hurdles, which we've presented in the briefest of ways, concerns the following. Are there gains to be made if the psychotherapy of schizophrenia is recast in part as the effort to help clients recover a greater capacity for dialogue? In our experience, there are, but only if one clears yet another hurdle. Helping people recover dialogical capacities requires the therapist to establish and carry on a dialogue with someone for whom dialogue is a primary problem. If schizophrenia, in both acute and post-acute phases of disorder, involves substantially weakened capacities to form and sustain intra- and interpersonal dialogues, how might deeply meaningful and transformative psychotherapeutic conversations occur? What steps are necessary for such a feat?

Before we address these questions, we wish to recount some previous efforts to explain how psychotherapeutic relationships form and work in schizophrenia. As noted, Karon and Van Denbos (1981) suggest that psychoanalytic knowledge enables the therapist to intuit underlying conflicts too painful for the client to realize – but this is problematic on two fronts. First, even if the observations were genuinely insightful, communicating and discussing them could remain problematic. One can have profound insights into others but remain trapped in a monologue about them if one is unable to genuinely discuss those observations and achieve some degree of mutual understanding about why the observation is insightful. Now, in this context, 'mutual understanding' does not entail identical understanding. As often happens between teacher and student, a student knows a portion of what the teacher knows, but with regard to that portion, both mutually understand it. Second, without some degree of mutual understanding about the practice and subject matter at hand, it is doubtful that the client will experience the purported insights as empathy. Although we find the language of 'mutual understanding' more precise than 'mutually constructed', we agree with Cohen (1996), who claims that in psychotherapy 'empathic connections are not as much a matter of perceiving the patient's experience as it is of mutually constructed shared narratives' (p. 614). Empathy has empowering effects because it overcomes feelings of isolation and provides recognition for one's understanding of one's situation. If mutual understanding is lacking, isolation will persist, and recognition never occur. We thus resist basing psychotherapeutic dialogue upon the epistemic privilege of the therapist.

Psychotherapy for schizophrenia thus faces the task of facilitating a conversation which arises in a shared space between two people (e.g., Atwood and Stoltorow, 1984; Mishara, 1995; Neimeyer, 1994). As Cohen and Schermer (2004) remark about psychoanalytic engagements, therapeutic relations arise and exist in an 'intersubjective field that the two parties construct' (p. 593). But how is this possible when dialogical compromise is the problem?

Psychotherapy through the lens of dialogism

In response to the question of whether dialogue is possible with people for whom having a dialogue is the problem, we will refrain from offering a single answer. Instead, each mode of compromised self-organization should be approached in its own manner, because each undermines dialogue in its own way. In what follows, we detail psychotherapeutic encounters with barren, monological, and cacophonous self-organizations, noting in each case the challenges each poses, and illustrating various steps that, when taken, seem to help clients recover dialogical capacity.

Note that as we discuss psychotherapy, we presume an 'integrative psychotherapy', that is, one that addresses, from multiple perspectives – for example, humanistic, psychodynamic, cognitive and constructivist traditions – how human beings make sense of their lives. The presumption is that the complexity of human dilemmas exceeds the purview of any single theory or set of psychotherapeutic methods. In each case, however, the perspectives employed are woven into an internally consistent network. Integrative psychotherapy consequently does not mean a haphazard application of techniques, but the ongoing integration of insights into a non-dogmatically defined, internally consistent perspective.

The actual psychotherapy that we discuss occurred weekly, was office-based, lasted 30 to 50 minutes, and took place under routine and voluntary conditions in an outpatient medical center in the mid-western United States. All clients were concurrently receiving antipsychotic medication which consisted of either one or two atypical agents taken orally. Several clients were prescribed mood-stabilizing medications as well. The dosages were all within the recommended ranges and there were few changes in dosing over the course of the psychotherapy discussed. As mentioned in the beginning of this volume, all identifying information including materials in quotes has been systematically disguised to protect confidentiality. Quoted material reflects prototypical comments and all names and other factual material within quotes have been systematically altered.

Integrative psychotherapy and barren self-organizations

Barren self-organizations pose difficult problems for therapists. Pieces of information emerge, but they never cohere into anything beyond the recitation of details. Moreover, clients of this sort do little to interpret and reflect upon the little they say. Recall Glass and his cloudbank. When asked what that meant, he seemed to think it was obvious: 'Whiteness in every direction.' Now, we are not suggesting that Glass was unable to speak about things. When asked, he related details about his day, but these were never presented or interpreted in relation to one another, or within the context of his pursuits and wishes. His remarks thus provided little sense about who he was as a person. As noted, one could infer character-positions from his remarks, but he never spoke of what it was like to be a brother, for example. It was as if the roles he played were minimal, skeletal structures for a minimal life.

The barrenness of Glass's self-organization manifests itself in another way that has bearings on his psychotherapy. He externalized all possible insight into his circumstances. When asked about what he thought was wrong, he suggested that 'doctors and nurses' knew, as well as his brother who had helped hospitalize Glass and who had seen him act in embarrassing ways. If asked what he thought about his belief that only others had insight into his own life, he replied: 'If I knew, I wouldn't be here.' That said, the externalized insights he occasionally encountered did not seem to improve his condition very much. He likened his initial sessions to 'skydiving without a parachute' and said he felt that he was hurtling 'downward' with 'nothing' to stop him. At the outset of his therapy, then, Glass presented himself as unable to adequately grasp or direct his life, but he also found little solace when handing these tasks over to health care professionals.

Psychotherapy may be especially difficult with those whose self-organization is barren because the client has little to say that the therapist might work with in order to facilitate the emergence of insight. In fact, clients may explicitly ask the therapist to do the work of presenting and synthesizing their lives. Glass often wanted his therapist to explain events in his life. With occasional annoyance and/or blank expressions, he repeatedly asked his therapist for an account of his own, i.e. Glass's, problems. On the one hand, such requests can be flattering, and one might be tempted to accept the challenges they pose. On the other hand, a client's persistent barrenness may prove disheartening. One may even take it to indicate one's own inadequacy as a therapist. If so, one might again feel tempted to provide one's client with some kind of life narrative in order to jump-start a life that has clearly foundered.

In our view, one should resist the temptation to give clients the story of their own life, and that includes a story like 'your flat affect is a negative symptom of a biologically based illness'. Not that those observations are forbidden, but they shouldn't form the heart of one's therapeutic exchanges. Genuine dialogue is unlikely to form if the client's story has been supplied by the therapist, irrespective of whether the therapist's account is accurate. In fact, authoritative accounts of his fate would only confirm Glass's belief that he has no capacity for insight, and that such matters should be left to doctors and nurses. It is worth noting that addressing the other in this way may also re-entrench stigma, insofar as it performatively situates the client in a passive role. Finally, the effort to try and fill in the barrenness of a client's self-organization seems to miss the point that barrenness results more from incapacities to create life-narratives amid the interanimating play of self-positions than from a deficient amount of thematic material.

Our fear, then, is that an effort to provide someone like Glass with a life-narrative would have paradoxically reinforced his or her barrenness, but we also think that silence, i.e., just letting the client talk in the manner that he or she sees fit, risks a similar result. In a conversational setting, silence isn't neutral. It often conveys disengagement, and undermines the kind of trust that genuine sharing requires. Moreover, as a therapeutic strategy, it inevitably leads to the position 'client, heal thyself'.

What then can be said? We encourage attending to those resources available to the client. Even in a barren self-organization, one perceives events, if in a constricted capacity. Glass saw people and events take place. Likewise, he was capable of self-regard; he presented himself as metaphorically falling. Moreover, such clients have self-positions; it is just that they do not enter into a dialogically rich, interanimating play. For example, Glass exhibited basic communicative competence, and thus he could play the roles of speaker and addressee. He could also fulfill other basic role expectations, for example, relating to his therapist (self-as-client) and family (self-as-brother).

Given these recourses, we believe that the therapist's task is not to remain silent, but to explicitly and repeatedly notice the perceptions that Glass offers, no matter how minimal, and underscore that these perceptions were ones that Glass had experienced. One can accomplish this by emphasizing the second-person dimensions of therapeutic address: '*You* heard,' and '*You* are wondering.' Glass said that he watched television, so his therapist asked the question: 'What did *you* watch?' 'How did *you* come to watch that?' Or: 'Do *you* remember something about that?' And when Glass replies negatively, the therapist replies: '*You* watch TV and later nothing comes to mind about what *you* saw?'

We begin with these stresses upon the second-person for several reasons. First, they implicitly treat clients as participants in the course of their lives, which grants them recognition as being more than passive players. Second, these questions call for responses that ask clients to participate more robustly in the course of their lives. In other words, in order to answer the questions in ways that respond to the stress upon 'you', clients must try perceiving, initially by way of memory, what they have undergone. This not only offers them some training in active perception, but over time, it rearticulates the expectation, implicit in all communicative relations, that they should be able to articulate to themselves and others what they have seen and done, and why. Moreover, it may also serve as an enabling condition for the generation of meta-positions and large-scale life narratives.

Given the habitual nature of the dialogical self, repeatedly returning to everyday events with an emphasis on the second-person should allow gains to accumulate. As clients begin to offer more thorough accounts of their lives, they are essentially forced to realize that they (and not only the therapist) are capable of insight into their lives. One might even say that they find their 'I' in the structural entailments of the singular 'you' to which they respond. We say this in part because the contours of Glass's agency began to take shape amid precisely these kinds of exchanges, which enabled his therapist to explicitly pose the question: 'who is Glass, this perceiver of events?' Our claim then is that the use of an emphatic '*You* saw/thought/met/felt … ' may assist clients with barren self-organizations to regard themselves as people capable of insight into their surroundings, of being more than one lost in a cloudbank.

Whether a client's remarks are actually insightful is not the immediate therapeutic concern. Rather, the therapeutic focus should be on helping them perform the kind of self-relations that enable insight and plausible responses to ordinary questions about their lives. Once that has been accomplished, one can focus on clients as protagonists in the events they are recalling. This might begin with joint speculations about feelings and ideas regarding their experiences, as well as reasons for actions, followed by inquiry into whether those speculations matched those events. Once he proved capable of offering interpretations concerning his own life, Glass began developing ideas about the significance of what he witnessed, that is, about its meaning for a life that *he* was pursuing. One time he recalled a horse-drawn carriage he had seen over the weekend. While discussing what enabled this recollection, Glass realized that he had purposefully waited to see the horse because he liked horses. The therapist then observed: '*You* watched the horse and seeing the horse was important to *you*.' Glass recognized this as correct, thereby encountering himself in pursuit of something, as someone who likes horses (which is a nascent metaposition), and who is able to act on that sense of self.

Remarkably, finding himself as an agent in pursuit of something, namely, the enjoyment of horses, sparked an interanimating play among some of Glass's self-positions. Following his observation, Glass recalled riding horses at a grandparent's farm as a child, and he realized that, as a child, he felt that his grandfather really loved and valued him. He then cried and discussed the death of his grandfather, which presented him then and there with a loss that he had never mourned. He then spoke further about his fear of funerals in general, and of how he avoided grief. This remarkable turn of events suggests, we think, that treating clients as an active perceiver and doer in the course of their life can stimulate latent capacities for reflective intra- and interpersonal dialogue, as well as cultivate those capacities through practice.

Of course, clients may report self-experiences that reassert their powerlessness in the course of their lives. After significant gains, Glass once related that while at work, someone from another department began to make 'small talk' while he tried to solve a confusing problem. He reported that during that brief encounter and again here, in therapy, he did not know what to do or say or even what he felt or thought. He was again empty. The therapist then asked: 'What would I have felt, and what would I have done?' Glass was able to form clear answers to these questions, and once he did, he suddenly had thoughts about how he felt and how he might have handled that particular situation differently, which informed him, he reported, that maybe he knew more about himself than he originally guessed. We share this episode because it exemplifies another therapeutic technique one might use to stimulate dialogical processes. At times, clients with barren self-organization struggle to ascertain their own thoughts, feelings, and experiences, even after they have come to regard themselves as capable of insight. However, they may nevertheless be able to assume the perspective of the therapist, and imagine how he or she might have fared in that situation. Glass could think about intentions and affects in the second-person as long as the therapist was the subject. He might say to the therapist: 'You would feel…'. After imagining the therapist having those qualities or intentions, he could then apply them to himself, and generate a sense of his own experience by way of contrast.

Once clients with barren self-experience prove able to regard themselves as capable of insight into their own lives, and of being protagonists in those lives, it may become possible for the therapist and client to begin exploring larger life narratives and more elaborate senses of self. This practice requires cooperative reflections that connect and explore material from previous sessions. In other words, here a life narrative emerges within an interpersonal dialogue, and precisely by stimulating in the client a series of intrapersonal dialogues. Over time, Glass worked his way into these activities. At one point, he began to argue with himself about what it meant that he was 'uninvolved', which we take to entail the generation of a meta-position. Along the way, his observations engaged multiple self-positions, for example, character-positions like self-as-grandson and self-as-heterosexual, as well as meta-positions like self-as-resenting-authority. In this rich context, he discovered that he was a person who tended to withdraw and 'shut down', even as he wished to reconnect with family, and so self-as-uninvolved assumed a rich, multifaceted patina that reflected the welfare of an agent pursuing determinate goals. More importantly, it evidenced that through the course of his psychotherapy, Glass's dialogical capacities had appreciably broadened and deepened. He still experienced desperate confusion and fear, but he also was able to develop a compassionate view of himself as an active participant in a life of struggle which entailed a meta-positional self-regard that provided some ballast for his sense of self.

We should stress that even at this point of dialogical sophistication, Glass did not possess an extended personal narrative. For example, he still could not articulate a life narrative in which thoughts and feelings were integrated across broad stretches of time. Nevertheless, his once thoroughly barren self-organization had been replaced by ongoing attempts to actively find and make meaning in a life touched and still marked by schizophrenia. In place of the cloudbank that once enveloped his sense of self, he now presented himself as someone who longed for a romantic attachment and a rebirth of earlier creative efforts. Not that this marked the end of his therapy. However, now that he was able to hold mostly coherent discussions about a future that could emerge from *his* present, his therapy began to resemble the therapy of people without psychoses.

Concurrent with his improvements in therapeutic reflection, Glass forged considerably deeper ties with his family, moved into his own apartment, and formed a range of new friendships based around hobbies. Moreover, his negative symptoms, including blunted affect and lack of volition, seemed to improve significantly, and he returned to work. These kinds of improvement suggest, we think, that as Glass's capacity for reflective dialogue deepened, so did his ability to undergo the myriad pre-reflective dialogues that everyday life initiates and conducts. The claim is not that psychotherapy allowed him to figure out his life. Rather, psychotherapy empowered him to better pursue it, and on his own terms, that is, in and through narratives that he had fashioned and was now capable of refashioning with the ongoing help of regular therapy.

Integrative psychotherapy and dialogue with monological selves

Whereas barren self-organizations correlate with unstructured self-presentations devoid of comparative and synthetic moments, monological scenarios involve the overwhelming integration of life experience. In the self-presentation of clients of this sort, one or two themes over-interpret the details of worldly encounters as well as flatten the depth and contract the breadth of intra- and interpersonal dialogue. Recall Grieg. After reading about a political gathering, he insisted that it occurred because a television celebrity loved him. When people at the supermarket stared at him, it was because they knew celebrities loved him. Others were jealous of the attention he received, and so they plotted to kidnap him and leave him bound and gagged deep in the woods.

In cases like Grieg's, a therapist faces someone with a more or less singular and unquestionable explanation for everything. Under such conditions, therapeutic dialogue is unlikely to begin. Grieg repeats himself over and over, which leaves nothing for the therapist to say in reply. After a few minutes of this, a novice or even the best-trained therapist is anxious for the monologue to stop. Where a barren narrative may leave a therapist feeling inadequate, a non-stop monologue may engender anger. A therapist might feel ignored, as if his or her training and insights meant nothing in the face of the client's certitude.

In such scenarios, the temptation is thus to interrupt the monologue. The therapist might point out the absurdity of the client's beliefs, and support the point with an appeal to the socially sanctioned diagnosis. In effect, the interruption would take the form of: 'you're not loved by celebrities, you have schizophrenia'.

We resist this approach, because it replaces the client's distorted, first-person stance with a drama that omits the first-person altogether. Instead of regarding clients as people struggling to make sense of frightening thoughts and experiences, one presents the reflexive intimacy of their life as the by-product of causal interactions, for example, among compromised neurocognitive processes and/or overpowering social-forces. This troubles us for three reasons. First, it bypasses the issue of compromised dialogical processes instead of addressing and re-establishing them. Second, it effectively presents clients with a life narrative instead of helping them build one that includes and thus empowers their struggles with mental illness. Finally, because exclusively third-person life narratives disqualify clients from being agents in the course of their own mental illness, this approach may intensify the effects of stigma.

We want to underscore that our concern does not lie with the truth or falsity of the diagnosis, but with how it performatively situates clients within psychotherapy. A therapist could ignore the content of Grieg's implausible claims and inform him that he suffered from a brain disease that made it difficult to process complex emotions, adding that, whenever complex emotions occurred, anxious and fearful organism-positions arose that manifested themselves in feelings of persecution. Even if these accounts are accurate, they nevertheless remove clients from the story of their lives. Yes, they may make plain that clients are not responsible for becoming mentally ill, but they also seem to suggest that they are not in part responsible for the future course of their illness. In our view, this throws the baby out with bath water, and overlooks a site where something like the reciprocal reconstruction of agency can commence, namely, in the intra- and interpersonal dialogues wherein clients encounter themselves as beloved, besieged, and mentally ill.

Presuming that silence is not an option (for the same reasons we gave with regard to barren self-organizations), how should the therapist intervene? One cannot work with the substance of what the client perceives, for that would keep the exchange locked within monological frames. Instead, we think one should focus upon what it's like to undergo these feelings of persecution and/or grandeur, and again with an emphasis upon the second-person dimensions of one's own address (and for the same reason – it requires the client to participate in the therapeutic dialogue, and as someone who is irreducible to his or her symptoms). This understanding could be expressed as reflections about how specific thoughts take control and make it impossible for the client to think of anything else: '*You* can only think of ...' or '*You* are consumed by this ...'. By reflecting upon the weight of a tyrannical voice that dominates all of daily life, the therapist avoids addressing the epistemic standing of the delusion or obsessive theme. This gives the pair something to talk about that touches upon the monologue without openly denying its content or dissolving into its monodrama. Of course, clients might and probably will, from time to time, interpret the therapist's behavior through their monologue. In these moments, our suggestion is to stay the course and inquire after what it's like to feel this way.

As with barren self-organizations, persistent questioning might slowly allow clients to uncover an 'I' in the form in which they are addressed, i.e. the 'you'. Not that this awakens some genuine self who has been buried beneath delusions, but it does disclose to clients that they are the ones undergoing and emotionally interpreting a range of phenomena, which establishes a modicum of distance between them and their delusions. This may habituate clients to reflect upon what it is like to undergo delusions, which also would provide them with an experience site that is not simply a function of the monologue (i.e. self-as-persecuted or self-as-beloved). Said otherwise, we are suggesting that an insistent therapeutic address might lead clients to internalize the dialogical structure embodied in their relationship with their therapist.

While initially resistant to remarks that contradicted his delusions, Grieg could accept the observation that there were times when he could only think about being kidnapped, and that this led him to shut out whatever his therapist might be saying or doing. Moreover, in soliciting the feelings that this insistent thought evoked, many of which involved fear and frustration, the therapist was able to lead Grieg to the realization that he wanted a life beyond the one this monological outlook provided, which further distanced Grieg from the grip of his monologue.

After empathizing with clients about the tyranny of their monologues, which opens a bit of conversational space, a second phase may prove possible in which therapy assumes a more cognitive and less emotional focus. This may involve examining how a belief or stance is experienced – for example, as unquestionable – and then how such a conclusion or position was reached. Doubt may be reinforced and the evidence for and against particular beliefs may be weighed in the manner of cognitive behavior therapy for schizophrenia, which has been widely described by others (e.g., Tarrier *et al.*, 2000). From a dialogical perspective, the gains here are less a matter of correcting false beliefs, although that may occur, and more a matter of allowing clients to experience the diversity and complexity of their lives.

Initially, Grieg agreed that his monological thoughts overwhelmed him, but explained that this was because 'they are real'. As the conversation deepened and he spoke of how it felt to live in such a world, another view slowly emerged, however. Grieg said that his mind reached certain conclusions no matter what was happening around him, and often in particular contexts. More often than not, he felt alone and uncertain about how to engage others. And in those moments, 'that kind of [monological] thinking just gets started'. When he was feeling alone, angry, and 'unable to love', he reported that the beliefs that formed the core of his monologue helped him to 'calm down'. Note that Grieg was not reporting that these beliefs were delusions, but he was beginning to experience himself in a world where his delusions come and go, and in response to worldly scenarios that are not part of the delusional landscape. At this stage in Grieg's therapy, more than one or two self-positions are beginning to emerge in his self-presentations, for example, the meta-position 'self-as-lonely', a recurring organism-position, 'self-as-angry', and a variety of character-positions – 'self-as-client' and 'self-as-roommate'. The more general point, then, is that by pressing clients to consider the full context in which their delusions are embedded, the life that had been lost to their monologues begins to emerge, creating the space for broader and deeper play among self-positions.

Following the examination of specific beliefs, the therapy might inquire after the client's broader life beyond his or her monodrama, perhaps focusing upon the therapeutic relation itself given the trust and stability that most likely now characterize it. The goal of these interventions lies with animating even more self-positions in order to disclose to clients the breadth of their real lives. Later in his therapy, Grieg noted being angry with his therapist, 'even though there is no reason'. He explained that he often directed anger and jealousy towards others, including the therapist, whose lives were, in his words, 'fine'. He often reflected upon why it was that others who also suffered trauma-filled childhoods were not 'mentally ill'. In reflecting upon these general feelings of anger and jealously, other self-positions were animated, including the meta-position 'mentally ill', but also character-positions like self-as-son and self-as-brother.

At this stage of psychotherapy, we should again stress that delusions may very well persist, but they may occur without reducing the client's self-organization to a monologue. In fact, they may come to occupy one or more moments within that organization, for example, in the form of a meta-position that Grieg named 'mental illness'. Moreover, such moments can now enter into reflective dialogue with other moments. After Grieg and his therapist agreed that Grieg's monologue was oppressive, they also came to see that for the time being it was indispensable. Grieg asked his therapist: 'Wouldn't you believe it if you thought a special celebrity loved you?' The therapist noted: 'I might be tempted to hang onto it when I felt bad about myself.' And Grieg found that true of himself. Believing that he was loved by celebrities made him feel better when he felt that no one in his immediate surroundings cared if he lived or died. Also, beliefs of persecution provided an explanation for why others rejected him, which did not involve his being inadequate. These events are noteworthy because they showed that as his intra- and interpersonal dialogues broadened and deepened, Grieg began to live with his mental illness, to reflect upon it and find in himself resources that delimited its once totalizing might.

At this point, Grieg, like Glass, still had not acquired a thoroughly integrated personal narrative. It was possible for him and his therapist to jointly connect events without the intrusion of his monologue, but his life narrative lacked extensive dialogical movement across long periods of time, including the future. Nevertheless, where a monologue once had reigned, Grieg now found himself actively interpreting and pursuing a life touched by schizophrenia and other vicissitudes of fate, including loss, longing and desires. He could coherently describe the thoughts and feelings of others and the impact of his behavior on them. Whereas previously, thoughts about being praised by celebrities enveloped his sense of self, he now presented himself as someone who wanted to fit in but was easily angered when he felt rejected. These advanced stages did not mark the end of his therapy, but as with Glass, Grieg's greatly strengthened dialogical capacities enabled his therapy to resemble more closely the therapy of people without psychoses. Concurrent with these improvements, Grieg also forged considerably deeper ties with his family and became more active over time, and in social ways, for example, he established phone service and began to use the bus system without help from caretakers. Finally, his positive symptoms, including hallucinations, delusions, and unusual thoughts, also appeared to improve significantly.

Integrative psychotherapy and cacophonous selves

The third pattern of compromised self-organization that we have associated with schizophrenia is a cacophonous one, which presents the therapist with a client who says multiple things at once, with few connections apparent among emerging ideas. Moreover, contradictions are common and treated as if they were not contradictions. Recall Purcell. He could speak quickly and continuously, with apparent passion and conviction, but without much if any ascertainable coherence. He once complained about his housing, for instance, but it was impossible to discern even the most basic details of his situation including whether he had a roommate, or how he got from his boarding house to the clinic. Here is a particularly cacophonous excerpt from one session:

> I wouldn't know lifestyle demand … Lifestyle demand is irrelevant anymore to me, because the reason I say it's irrelevant is because the words are more important, and yet they decrease your style of living for the benefit that there's no bad actions, you know. That way you're liable to forget you see, and I can understand that, but if I wanted to put something intact this immediate, it would be mine.

Because Purcell's speech is so disordered, and to the point that it is difficult to find expressive meaning in what he says (though less so in how he says it, at least for those present), one could imagine concluding either that (a) psychotherapy is impossible under such conditions, or (b) that one should supply a structure for discussion.

In their disorder, cacophonous self-organizations, like barren and monological self-organizations, can tempt a therapist to supply clients with ordered life narratives. Even if they do not, an aligned risk nevertheless confronts the therapist. In the chaos of the client's speech, it will be tempting to find one's own cherished struggles and meanings at play in the client's scattered yet suggestive remarks, for example, loneliness, struggles with social oppression, evidence of familial unhappiness, etc. It's as if a cacophonous self-presentation becomes an inkblot for the therapist's own life dramas. In any case, no matter how accurate or absurd one's intuitions prove, projecting them usurps the client's life narrative and leaves their dialogical compromises unaddressed.

Presuming again that silence offers little support, in cases like these we suggest an intervention that continuously reflects or mirrors whatever clients reveal about themselves, which may involve allowing the client to move from disclosure to disclosure without protest or effort to connect them. Here the emphasis is not upon 'You perceived X', as in the case of barren self-organizations. Rather, one relies upon observations like, 'You are …' and/or 'You are feeling …'. The approach is thus similar to what we suggested regarding monological self-organizations, but with less of an exclusively affective focus. The notion here is that within the client's cacophonous speech are fragments of self-positions. The therapist's initial task is thus to notice, reinforce and support those fragments as they arise and, as we've suggested throughout this chapter, ensuring that the second-person of one's address is heard may provide clients, within the therapeutic exchange (if not elsewhere as well), with a greater reflexive orientation towards their behavior.

It is important to underscore that in cacophonous self-organizations, self-disclosures are often buried in third-person generalizations, and with very few if any apparent character-positions. Observing and highlighting emerging self-positions thus often requires the therapist to venture working translations of client remarks, with a focus upon organism and meta-positions. Purcell once said something to the effect of 'people in general are angry and not to be trusted'. In reply, the therapist noted: 'You're angry', and then 'You are not to be trusted.' Shortly thereafter there were comments that the therapist could not follow, followed by the claim that people in general shun the wounded, to which the therapist replied, 'You are shunned.' Purcell then said: 'The head of the body is in pain.' And the therapist said in return: 'You have a headache.' Note that, excepting these personalizing translations, the self-presentations are left as is. At this stage, no attempt is made to construct any larger state of affairs, such as: 'You are angry because you feel you have been shunned, and now have a headache.'

Given our dialogical lens, this initial work with cacophonous clients seems to involve strengthening self-positions. Each time a self-position is correctly identified it seems to gather strength until, at some point, it has its own standing – self-as-angry, self-as-brother, self-as-shunned. In our view, the binding agent lies in habituation and the intersubjective recognition provided by the therapist. In the therapist's affirmation of recurring thoughts and feelings (and the self-positions to which they are tied), clients recognize self-facets as *their* facets. Initially, Purcell seemed reassured by each 'You feel …' statement, and in time he began to appear generally more coherent. Yet he virulently resisted empathy from the therapist and spoke almost exclusively in abstract riddles for much of the first year. Recalling our previous discussion of psychosocial dysfunction, it was as if empathy set an overwhelming intersubjective presence within Purcell's self-organization, whereas less personal observations of his self-presentations proved bearable.

Once self-positions begin to emerge, and clients make more statements about how they feel, a two-part, second phase emerges, which requires the synthesis of self-presentations. On the one hand, the therapist tries to help the client connect self-presentations. On the other hand, he or she seeks out presentations of the worldly contexts within which these self-positions arose. The thought here is that each task is mutually supportive. Self-positions, worldly by nature, bring with them context-rich scenarios, and these scenarios suggest additional self-positions, and so on. In short, the goal is to recall the full, intra- and interpersonal world eclipsed by surging cacophonies.

At one point, Purcell remarked: 'No one can get along in this world.' The therapist replied: 'You can't get along in this world.' Purcell seemed to agree, but kept to the universal. 'When people try, it all goes bad.' As you might now guess, the therapist suggested, bringing together a series of remarks: 'You think that, if you try to get along, it will all go bad, and people will shun you.' Interestingly, at this point, Purcell laughed giddily and said, 'Yeah, that's right.' 'Why?' the therapist asked. Purcell proceeded to contextualize the mutually constructed observation, bringing together several previous disclosures within a more coherent life narrative centered on feelings of abandonment. He recalled how relatives had raised him away from his siblings and how he was angry at having been separated in this way. At the time, he felt as if his surrogate parents hadn't really loved him, although he now confessed to perhaps not having given them a chance, particularly since he had come to learn that the grandmother who raised him had also struggled with mental illness. While discussing these things, he observed that the therapist reminded him of his parole officer from the period they were discussing, namely high school, but he did so in keeping with the theme of abandonment, for this man had been married to a woman who taught him art until she left school to marry the principal. We find this exchange remarkable because it shows Purcell beginning to present himself, in the both the past and present, as an agent in his own life, and in a way that broadens and deepens as the story is told. Moreover, once it leaves the abstract generalizations behind, the tale evidences multiple self-positions, for example, self-as-sibling, self-as-grandson, self-as-student, self-as-parolee, self-as-abandoned, self-as-hurt, self-as-fearful, etc., and in ways that interanimate one another. Of course, there is still pain, but Purcell is presenting it as *his* pain within a plausible self-narrative whose protagonist he was and remains.

At this juncture, it is worth noting that Purcell sometimes needed to approach his own life narrative indirectly. At times, he personalized his generalizations, but with the therapist as their subject. He would attribute to the therapist various sexual desires or strong emotions, to which the therapist would say: 'You see me as a sex maniac', or, 'You see me as a very angry person.' In other words, the therapist would not contradict Purcell; just clarify the source of the attribution. Over time, Purcell would begin to internalize these projections, and set them within his larger life story of abandonment, abuse, hospitalization, etc. As in the case of barren self-organizations, it would seem that clients can better apprehend their own polyphonic life story if the protagonist is first someone else, as if it's initial complexity were easier to bear when set upon someone else's shoulders. Regardless, once this turn back towards the self is made, richly contextualized life scenarios begin to unfold, as we saw above.

Purcell, for instance, sometimes called the therapist 'kind', 'angry', 'stupid', and 'dangerous'. He went on to accuse the therapist of deep envy and greed and a secret wish to harm others. Here the therapist did not say, for instance, 'You are envious and greedy...'. Instead the response was 'You know how people can have greed and envy...'. Over the next year, subject to these kinds of redirections, Purcell began to interiorize these very same states and with striking clarity. He began to not only express different self-positions but to reflect on their relation. He noted that he was 'paying the price of not caring for myself for years'. He also noted that he sought 'connection with others' but feared ridicule, and that he was 'too hard' on himself. His therapist once said, 'You are the king of self neglect.' Purcell laughed and proceeded, more or less with himself, to discuss what it would take to give that up as a lifestyle.

We wish to stress that the added coherence in Purcell's self-presentation did not follow from his reception of a skeletal life narrative, courtesy of his therapist. Instead, the therapist would preserve and set beside one another various self-attributions. In other words, the therapist would facilitate the beginnings of dialogical movement among self-positions, as well as among their attendant thoughts and feelings. From this, Purcell became more adept at conceiving of and presenting himself as the protagonist of his own life story.

Improvement does not indicate a full return to well-being, however. Like Grieg and Glass, Purcell has not acquired a thoroughly integrated personal narrative, and the coherence of his self-presentations can fluctuate. Nevertheless, Purcell has left behind the sheer incoherence of his initial, cacophonous self-presentations. Moreover, he has reached a point where limited but coherent dialogue is possible, both in therapy and beyond its relatively safe walls. Whereas previously a spray of unrelated verbalizations enveloped his sense of self, he became someone who presented himself as intentionally rejecting the world rather than waiting to be rejected by it again.

Summary

In this chapter, we have suggested that a dialogical account of the self may help us think differently about the goals and even technical requirements of an integrative psychotherapeutic approach to schizophrenia. In particular, we think that psychotherapy for schizophrenia should in part be understood as an effort to reignite intra- and interpersonal dialogue. The hope is that by empowering dialogical capacities, clients will cease to experience themselves as sites of diminishment and regain the sense that they are dynamic centers of insight and action.

At the level of technique, a dialogically informed psychotherapy for schizophrenia should take into account how the client's self-organization has been compromised by schizophrenia. The thought is that each mode of self-organization requires somewhat different treatment, even though certain techniques are appropriate for all. On the whole, the rule is, begin with whatever dialogical resources are available to the client. With clients suffering from barren self-organizations, the therapist should focus upon their ability to perceive and recall the world of their experience, cultivating it, and then focus on ways in which clients are protagonists within the events they perceive. Because monological self-organizations are characterized by delusional perceptions, in these instances, therapy instead should provide empathic observations of the affects such perceptions provoke. The goal is similar, however: namely, to disclose to clients that, despite the apparent unquestionable authority of these thoughts, they nevertheless have their own affective responses to them, responses that often indicate a desire to live in non-monological ways. Building in the spaces that experience evidences, the therapist can then employ the techniques of cognitive behavior therapy to further weaken the grip of delusions and allow clients to experience them as contextualized phenomena with which they can cope. Finally, with those caught in cacophonous self-organizations, the therapist should collect and present whatever clients reveal about themselves, which may require the therapist to translate universal statements ('people are angry') into particular ones ('you are angry'). The goal here is to help clients find themselves within whatever self-positions quickly enter into and disappear from their self-presentations. The next step involves mutually constructing a narrative that weaves these self-positions and the contexts of their emergence into a life that clients recognize as their own.

While these approaches to different modes of self-organization are notable, they should be viewed as additions to a more basic dialogical approach to psychotherapy for schizophrenia. At its most general, an integrative psychotherapy for schizophrenia, pursued through the lens of dialogism, wishes neither to provide clients with surrogate life narratives, nor remain silent in the presence of their self-presentations. If dialogical processes are going to be sparked and strengthened, their first-person dimensions must be recognized and cultivated. This is pursued in part through re-presenting the self-presentations of clients in order that they might be able to encounter and respond to that disclosure more richly than was previously possible. In order to keep clients focused upon their own place in and contribution to the fates they describe, the therapist should address clients with a stress upon the second-person aspect of their remarks, namely, the 'you' who might be attending a basketball game, feeling angry, or struggling with a roommate. The stress invites clients into the therapeutic dialogue, and as another 'I'. As we argued in Chapter 3, communication builds upon our organism's reflexive capacities, instituting a reflective dimension within character-positions, and enabling us to pursue the more general activity of reflective dialogue. A therapeutic stress upon the second-person, which continually references thoughts, feelings, and actions to the client, repeats that building process in an effort to expand the first-person capacities of clients, both in and beyond the therapeutic setting.

As the process of deepening and broadening dialogical processes evolves, the therapist continues to respect the first-person dimensions of the client's plight by remaining oriented towards a mutual understanding of the basic concepts that organize emerging life narratives. In other words, the expert language of systematic psychology is not allowed to tell clients who they are. Instead, they are encouraged to articulate their own sense of self as it is disclosed to them in the reflections that therapy enables, as well as through the course of their lives. Of course, like everyone, clients will rely upon terms that they did not generate *ex nihilo*, but that reliance will be one that they grow into through sustained reflection.

We should stress that we are in no way suggesting that dialogical theory can turn psychotherapy into a 'cure' for schizophrenia. Rather, the goal is to enable people to live effectively with their illness, the threat of stigmatization, and the like. Our claim is that (a) improved dialogical capacities should allow people with schizophrenia to address their illness and its attendant problems in a manner that approximates how others address problems when psychosis isn't present, and (b) that dialogically inflected psychotherapy for schizophrenia helps brings this about. We claim the latter because in all three of the cases discussed, the clients in question, namely, Grieg, Glass, and Purcell, experienced, over the course of their therapy, decreases in symptoms, improved psychosocial functioning, and the re-emergence of a sense that they were something of a protagonist in the course of their lives. Not that problems did not persist, including symptoms associated with schizophrenia, which merited continued treatment, but having those problems ceased to be the sole, defining feature of their lives, or of whom they took themselves to be.

Chapter 8

Conclusion

Summary

Our initial chapters reviewed two bodies of literature regarding schizophrenia. After outlining its basic features, Chapter 1 addressed prevailing theories about the biological and social forces that significantly contribute to the onset and course of the illness. With regard to these theories, we argued that for all their power they tend to neglect the first-person dimensions of schizophrenia, namely, how the symptoms and challenges posed by the illness are disclosed to, interpreted by, and ultimately lived with by human beings. Chapter 2 gathered from diverse theoretical perspectives some commonly observed, first-person aspects of schizophrenia. Drawing these observations into a single portrait, we found people with widespread experiences of diminishment, for example, with regard to social relationships or strong emotions, who had a sense of themselves as broken, even absorbed by their own mental illness.

Our principal concern, then, has been articulating and exploring the first-person dimensions of schizophrenia. More specifically, we've considered how people come to experience themselves as diminishing over the course of their illness, sometimes quite profoundly. We have also considered the impact of such experiences upon a wide range of symptoms as well as social and vocational disability. However, before pursuing these concerns, we tried to account for how sense of self arises for anyone. In Chapter 3, we argued that sense of self does not involve the apprehension of a substantial self that resides within us. Instead, we sense ourselves within and through dialogues that are bound to worldly interactions, at once intra- and interpersonal, and that reflect complementary and dissonant facets of our being. More precisely, sense of self emerges out of an interaction among self-positions, namely, character-positions, organism-positions, and meta-positions. Properly speaking, character and organism-positions are not judgments about ourselves. Rather, they are more or less habitual axes of self–world interaction wherein the character and welfare of our being is disclosed to us, and while meta-positions do arise in reflective, self-presentations, they come to function in ways that exceed the phenomenon of judgment. Our overall claim, then, is that sense of self is dialogical, the disclosure of a being to itself through an interanimating play of multiple, often partially discontinuous self-facets within shifting worldly contexts.

Having provided an account of sense of self and how it emerges, we returned in Chapter 4 to see if disruptions in dialogical processes could account for the kinds of self-experiences that clinicians and researchers, over the last hundred years, have associated with schizophrenia. We argued that dialogical compromises contribute to the experience of self-diminishment that often accompanies the appearance of schizophrenia. Moreover, since compromises of this kind do not fully undermine one's ability to sense one's self, we also suggested that approaching experiences of self-disruption through dialogical compromise could account for how people are both diminished and able to recognize it. Such an account is useful because it both clarifies and helps explain a neglected facet of schizophrenia, and in a manner that preserves the first-person dimensions of the illness. Moreover, it does so in a way that helps synthesize observations from diverse theoretical perspectives.

Chapter 4 also suggested that a model of dialogical compromise could lead to at least three different forms of diminished self-experience: a self experienced as a cacophony, as a barren and empty landscape, and as a monologue where life is dominated by a single view. We consider these models useful additions to the literature on schizophrenia because they refine our feel for what it is like to live with schizophrenia, and they help us distinguish some markedly different ways in which someone's sense of self can be undermined over the course of the illness.

In Chapter 5, we asked whether a dialogical account of schizophrenia could help us understand the emergence of symptoms, or whether, while preserving schizophrenia's first-person dimensions, it led to a kind of dualism. In reply, we suggested that several characteristic symptoms (complex verbal hallucinations, systematized delusions, blunted affect, lack of volition, and poor insight) might exacerbate and be exacerbated by dialogical compromises. Our claim then is that, while symptoms and self-experience may be distinct in schizophrenia, they may also mutually affect one another via the thread of dialogical disturbance.

In Chapter 6, we considered whether compromises in dialogical capacities might play a role in psychosocial dysfunction. We have argued that social forces, which lead to dysfunction such as stigma and oppressive power relationships, may exacerbate and be exacerbated by dialogical compromises. We further argued that intersubjectivity, because it animates dialogical processes, and in unpredictable ways, may undermine already weakened dialogical orders. As a result, social life may be experienced as a threat and intimacy avoided, two effects that in turn seem to intensify dialogical breakdowns, which could lead to a debilitating downward spiral. Finally, we suggested that the dialogical demands of committed action also bring disorder to dialogical processes among people with schizophrenia, thereby possibly leading them to avoid or have difficulties sustaining commitment.

Taken together, Chapters 5 and 6 also suggest that a dialogical approach to schizophrenia gives us reason to suppose that first-person dimensions interact with third-person events over the course of the illness. In the cases of positive and negative symptoms, as well as psychosocial dysfunction, we have witnessed some of the ways in which self-disclosures, in the form of dialogue among self-positions, might render one vulnerable to and intensify the effects of oppressive social relationships, cognitive deficits, abnormal cortical activity, and so forth. These two chapters thus provide some reasons to believe the claim that how one experiences, interprets and lives with schizophrenia is relevant to how it unfolds over the course of one's life.

Our final chapter argues that dialogism has implications for how one might pursue individual psychotherapy for schizophrenia. We should stress that we are in no way suggesting that dialogical theory can turn psychotherapy into a "cure" for schizophrenia. Rather, our goal is to enable people to live effectively with their illness and its attendant difficulties. Our claim, then, is that improved dialogical capacities, which a dialogically inflected psychotherapy facilitates, should allow people with schizophrenia to address their illness as others address problems when psychosis is not present.

Limitations

While we find these lines of inquiry promising, they are limited in ways that should be kept in mind. First, while our study draws from years of clinical experience and research, its empirical basis has been limited to a few settings with a limited number and certain type of client. We consequently do not know how our view would have changed or will change if and when we engage different kinds of people in different locales and contexts, for example, people who refuse treatment, women, or people of color.

We have also only been able to provide a truncated presentation of our theory of self-experience. Given that our principal focus has been diminished self-experience in schizophrenia, there were many questions that we could not address without writing two books under one cover. Moreover, our theoretical palette is an admittedly broad one, for example, existential phenomenology, pragmatic social theory, Nietzsche, Bahktin, and contemporary dialogical theory as developed by Hermans and others. Undoubtedly, many readers would like to know more about what we took and did not take from these thinkers and traditions. Unfortunately, attending to issues would have required yet a third study, and so we elected to present, in more or less our own terms, a hopefully coherent, synthesized view. Finally, there are also several well-developed positions that bear on our view, but which we could not engage and still maintain our focus on first-person experience in schizophrenia.

Additionally, while addressing the so-called traditional hallmarks of schizophrenia, we were only able to focus on five out of a whole host of symptoms. Not addressed, but likely relevant to diminished self-experience, are symptoms related to anxiety, depression, lack of inhibition and hyperarousal. We also did not discuss the possible interface of declines or improvements in cognitive capacity with evolving changes in dialogical capacity. Is dialogical capacity more imperiled, for instance, by fundamental failures to encode and organize basic sensory input or by the degradation of higher order functions which allow for inhibition and mental flexibility?

Finally, our discussion of individual integrative psychotherapy is far from and not meant to be a "perfected" (let alone exclusive) method of treatment. Other psychotherapeutic techniques or therapeutic activities may also help people recover dialogical capacities, and we have not pursued the full range of possible engagements available, nor discussed them. Second, the treatments presented involved various medications, and there may be other, more effective agents, some of which have yet to be discovered or tested. We've also only discussed clients in individual psychotherapy. Group psychotherapy, which was not discussed here, also seems to offer clients conversations that might enrich dialogical capacity.

Future directions

Measurement and assessments

Taken as a whole, our project is as much a beginning as a result, but it is a determinate beginning that suggests future research projects. First, we are interested in developing and refining tools to assess dialogical capacity. To avoid the fatal end point of being yet another unverifiable theory, we see the need to find ways to measure dialogical capacity in schizophrenia. To that end we have begun to gather the personal narratives of people with schizophrenia, and we are actively trying to create reliable means of assessing the presence and variety of self-positions within those narratives.

With assessments of these phenomena, we expect to be able to correlate dialogical capacity and diversity with a range of other quantitative measures including various domains of neurocognition, objective assessments of symptoms and internalized stigma. For instance, we seek to develop methods that will allow us to test whether assessments of dialogical capacity within a narrative sample are linked with observable behavioral and social deficits. This work may also possibly bear on the issue of whether different pharmaceutical agents, particularly those touted to enhance cognition, have differential effects on dialogical capacity and self-experience. For instance, do some medications have special value when it comes to assisting people to recover lost dialogical capacity?

Self-positions, temporality and praxis

In addition to these empirical questions, there is much more to say about and in defense of the dialogical self (as noted in our limitations section). Other topics of concern include our temporality. This seems an obvious pre-condition for self-relation in general, but it is uncertain how one might account for it in a way that keeps it a temporality of particular human beings-in-the-world, which preserves the first-person dimensionality of our temporalized nature. We would also like to explore how self-positions, and not just organism-positions, are embodied. One has to wonder how the praxical competencies of self-positions are enabled by and inform the competencies of our bodily comportment. Gaining a foothold in this latter issue might then enable us to consider how people with schizophrenia experience themselves as disembodied.

Psychosocial rehabilitation

Finally, while we have discussed individual psychotherapy at length, we have not explored psychosocial rehabilitation, a group of treatments that seek to help people engage or re-engage in basic community activities. Examples of psychosocial interventions include vocational programs such as supported employment, which helps people return to competitive work, club houses, which offer people peer support and guidance, and case management, which provides active outreach to people who might otherwise have difficulties supporting themselves.

In general, rehabilitation programs seek to advocate for the needs of disabled people and assist them to access opportunities they may have been denied. We are particularly keen to explore them because they are currently the treatments of choice for people with schizophrenia, and because they seem intimately bound to dialogical phenomena. In particular, psychosocial rehabilitation involves social situations that inevitably elicit and interpolate self-positions, some of which will prove novel for the clients involved. It would seem, then, that a client's relative dialogical capacity would be relevant to his or her experiences and success in whatever program he or she pursues. Attending to issues of dialogical incapacity and diminished self-experience may therefore help practitioners better understand the full range of challenges that psychosocial rehabilitation poses for people with schizophrenia, including persistence in the program and the integration of program experiences into larger, future oriented, life-narratives.

References

Amador, X. F., Flaum, M., Andreasen, N., Strauss, D. H., Yale, S. A., Clark, S. C. *et al.* (1994). Awareness of illness in schizophrenia and mood disorders. *Archives of General Psychiatry*, *51*(10), 826–836.

American Psychiatric Association (2000). *Diagnostic and statistical manual of mental disorders* (4th edn, text revision). Washington, DC: American Psychiatric Association.

Andreasen, N. C., Arndt, S., Swayze, V., Cizadlo, T., Flaum, M., O'Leary, D. *et al.* (1994). Thalamic abnormalities in schizophrenia visualized through magnetic image averaging. *Science*, *266*, 294–298.

Andreasen, N. C., Flaum, M., Swayze, V. W., Tyrrell, G. and Arndt, S. (1990). Positive and negative symptoms in schizophrenia: A critical reappraisal. *Archives of General Psychiatry*, *47*, 615–621.

Asarnow, J. R., Thompson, M. C. and McGrath, E. P. (2004). Childhood onset schizophrenia: Clinical and treatment issues. *Journal of Child Psychology and Psychiatry*, 45, 180–194.

Atwood, G. and Stolorow, R. (1984). *Structures of subjectivity: Explorations in psychoanalytic phenomenology*. Hillsdale, NJ: Analytic Press.

Bachrach, L. L. (1992). What we know about homelessness among mentally ill persons: An analytical review and commentary. *Hospital and Community Psychiatry*, *43*, 453–464.

Bak, R. C. (1954). The schizophrenic defense against aggression. *International Journal of Psychoanalysis*, *35*, 129–134.

Bakhtin, M. (1985). *Problems of Dostoyevsky's poetics* (C. Emerson, trans.). Minneapolis, MN: University of Minnesota Press. (Original work published 1929).

Barham, P. (1993). *Schizophrenia and human value*. London: Free Association Books.

Beck, A. T., Rush, A. J., Shaw, B. F. and Emery, G. (1979). *Cognitive therapy of depression*. New York: Guilford Press.

Benjamin, L. S. (1989). Is chronicity a function of the relationship between the person and the auditory hallucination? *Schizophrenia Bulletin*, *15*, 291–310.

Bhugra, D. (2000). Migration and schizophrenia. *Acta Psychiatrica Scandinavica* Supplement, 407, 68–73.

Bion, W. R. (1967). *Second thoughts*. New York: Jason Aronson.

Birchwood, M., Meaden, A., Trower, P., Gilbert, P. and Plaistow, J. (2000). The power and omnipotence of voices: Subordination and entrapment by voices and significant others. *Psychological Medicine*, *30*, 337–334.

Blankenburg, W. (2001). First steps toward a psychopathology of 'common sense.' *Philosophy*, *Psychology* and *Psychiatry*, *8*, 303–315.

Bleuler, E. (1950). *Dementia praecox or the group of schizophrenias* (J. Zinkin, trans.). New York: International Universities Press. (Original work published 1911).

Bond, G. R., Drake, R. E., Mueser, K. T. and Becker, D. R. (1997). An update of supported employment for people with severe mental illness. *Psychiatric Services*, *48*(3), 335–346.

Bordieri, J. E. and Drehmer, D. E. (1986). Hiring decision for disabled workers: Looking at the cause. *Journal of Applied Social Psychology*, *16*(3), 197–208.

Boss, M. (1979). *Existential foundations of medicine and psychology* (S. Conway and A. Cleaves, trans.). New York: Jason Aronson.

Bovet, P. and Parnas, J. (1993). Schizophrenia delusions: A phenomenological approach. *Schizophrenia Bulletin*, *19*, 579–597.

Bowie, C. R., Tsapelas, I., Friedman, J., Parrella, M., White, L. and Harvey, P. D. (2005). The longitudinal course of thought disorder in geriatric patients with chronic schizophrenia. *American Journal of Psychiatry*, *162*(4), 793–795.

Braff, D. L. (1993). Informational processing and attention dysfunctions in schizophrenia. *Schizophrenia Bulletin*, *19*, 233–259.

Breier, A., Buchanan, R. W., Elkashef, A., Munson, R. C. and Gellad, F. (1992). Brain morphology and schizophrenia: A magnetic resonance imaging study of limbic, prefrontal cortex and caudate structures. *Archives of General Psychiatry*, *49*(12), 921–926.

Brenner, C. A., Sporns, O., Lysaker, P. H. and O'Donnell, B. F. (2003). EEG synchronization to modulated auditory tones in schizophrenia, schizoaffective disorder and schizotypal personality disorder. *American Journal of Psychiatry*, *160*, 2238–2240.

Bryson, G., Bell, M. and Lysaker, P. H. (1997). Affect recognition in schizophrenia: A function of global impairment or a specific cognitive deficit. *Psychiatry Research*, *71*, 105–113.

Calasso, R. (1994). *The Marriage of Cadmus and Harmony* (T. Parks, trans.). New York: Vintage International.

Carter, M. and Flesher, S. (1995). The neurosociology of schizophrenia: Vulnerability and functional disability. *Psychiatry*, *58*, 209–221.

Chadwick, P. and Birchwood, M. (1994). The omnipotence of voices: A cognitive approach to auditory hallucinations. *British Journal of Psychiatry*, *164*, 190–201.

Chua, S. E. and McKenna, J. J. (1995). Schizophrenia: A brain disease? A critical review of structural and functional cerebral abnormality in the disorder. *British Journal of Psychiatry*, *165*, 563–582.

Clementz, B. A. and Sweeney, J. A. (1990). Is eye movement dysfunction a biological marker for schizophrenia? A methodological review. *Psychological Bulletin*, *108*, 77–92.

Cohen, M. C. (1996). Schizophrenia, perception and empathy. *Journal of the American Academy of Psychoanalysis*, *23*, 603–617.

Corrigan, P. W. (2003). Toward an integrated structural model of psychiatric rehabilitation. *Psychiatric Rehabilitation Journal, 26,* 346–358.

Corrigan, P. W. and Penn, D. L. (1999). Lessons from social psychology on discrediting psychiatric stigma. *American Psychologist, 54,* 765–775.

Coursey, R. D., Keller, A. B. and Farrell, E. W. (1995). Individual psychotherapy and persons with severe mental illness: The client's perspective. *Schizophrenia Bulletin, 21,* 283–301.

Cuffel, B. J., Alford, J., Fischer, E. P. and Owen, R. R. (1996). Awareness of illness in schizophrenia and outpatient treatment adherence. *Journal of Nervous and Mental Disease, 184*(11), 653–659.

Damasio, A. R. (1999). *The feeling of what happens.* New York: Putman.

David, A. S. (1994). The neuropsychological origin of auditory hallucinations. In A. S. David and J. C. Cutting (eds), *The neuropsychiatry of schizophrenia* (pp. 269–313). Mahwah, NJ: Lawrence Erlbaum.

Davidson, L. (2003). *Living outside mental illness: Qualitative studies of recovery in schizophrenia.* New York: New York University Press.

Davidson, L. and Stayner, D. (1997). Loss, loneliness and the desire for love: Perspectives on the social lives of people with schizophrenia. *Psychiatric Rehabilitation Journal, 20,* 3–12.

Davies, P., Thomas, P. and Leudar, I. (1999). Dialogical engagement with voices: A single case study. *British Journal of Medical Psychology, 27,* 179–187.

Davis, L. W. and Lysaker, P. H. (2005). Cognitive behavioral therapy and functional and metacognitive outcomes in schizophrenia: A single case study. *Cognitive and Behavioral Practice, 12,* 468–478.

Delisi, L. E., Sakuma, M., Tew, W., Kushner, M., Hoff, A. L. and Grimson, R.(1997). Schizophrenia as a chronic active brain process: A study of progressive brain structural change subsequent to the onset of schizophrenia. *Psychiatry Research, 74,* 120-140.

Dewey, J. (1988). *Human nature and conduct.* In: *The middle works of John Dewey:* Vol. 14. Carbonodale, IL: Southern Illinois University Press. (Original work published 1922).

Dickerson, F. B., Sommerville, J., Origoni, A. E., Ringel, R. B. and Parente, F. E. (2002). Experiences of stigma among outpatients with schizophrenia. *Schizophrenia Bulletin, 28,* 143–147.

Dostoyevsky, F. (1993) *Crime and punishment.* New York: Alfred A. Knopf. (Original work published 1866).

Drake, R. E. and Sederer, L. I. (1986). The adverse effects of intensive treatment of schizophrenia. *Comprehensive Psychiatry, 27,* 313–326.

Drury, V., Birchwood, M., Cochrane, R. and MacMillian, F. (1996). Cognitive therapy and recovery from acute psychosis: A controlled trial. *British Journal of Psychiatry,169,* 593–601.

Emerson R. W. (1964). In: Whicher, S., Spiller, R. E. and Williams, W. (eds), *The early lectures of Ralph Waldo Emerson: Volume II, 1836–1838*. Cambridge, MA: Harvard University Press.

Estroff, S. E. (1989). Self, identity and subjective experiences of schizophrenia. *Schizophrenia Bulletin, 15*(2), 189–196.

Fenton, W. S. (2000). Evolving perspectives on individual psychotherapy for schizophrenia. *Schizophrenia Bulletin, 26*, 47–72.

Flanagan, O. (1994). Multiple identity, character transformation and self-reclamation. In G. Graham and G. L. Stephens (eds), *Philosophical Psychopathology* (pp. 135–162). Cambridge, MA: The MIT Press.

Francis, J. L. and Penn, D. L. (2001). The relationship between insight and social skills in persons with severe mental illness. *Journal of Nervous and Mental Disease, 189*, 822–829.

Frankel, B. (1993). Groups for the chronic mental patient and the legacy of failure. *International Journal of Group Psychotherapy, 43*, 157–172.

Freud, S. (1957). Neurosis and psychosis (A. Strachey and J. Strachey, trans.). *Collected papers, Vol. II*. London, England: Hogarth Press.

Fromm-Reichmann, F. (1954). Psychotherapy of schizophrenia. *American Journal of Psychiatry, 111*, 410–419.

Frosh, J. (1983). *The psychotic process*. New York: International Universities Press.

Fucetola, R., Seidman, L. J., Kremen, W. S., Faraone, S. V., Goldstein, S. J. and Tsuang, M. T. (2000). Age and neurologic function in schizophrenia: A decline in executive abilites beyond that observed in healthy volunteers. *Biological Psychiatry, 48*, 137–146.

Gadamer, H. G. (1981). *Reason in the age of science*. Cambridge, MA: MIT University Press.

Gallese, V. (2001). The 'shared manifold' hypothesis: From mirror neurons to empathy. *Journal of Consciousness Studies, 8*(5–7), 33–50.

Gilbert, P., Birchwood, M., Gilbert, J., Trower, P., Hay, J., Murray, B. *et al.* (2001). An exploration of evolved mental mechanisms for dominant and subordinate behavior in relation to auditory hallucinations in schizophrenia and critical thoughts in depression. *British Journal of Medical Psychology, 31*, 1117–1127.

Glover, J. (2001). Psychiatric disorder and the reactive attitudes. *Public Affairs Quarterly, 15*, 291–307.

Goff, D. C., Cather, C., Evins, A. E., Henderson, D. C., Freudenreich, O., Copeland *et al.* (2005). Medical morbidity and mortality in schizophrenia: Guidelines for psychiatrists. *Journal of Clinical Psychiatry, 66*, 183–194.

Goffman, E. (1963). *Stigma: Notes on the management of spoiled identity*. Englewood Cliffs, NJ: Prentice-Hall.

Gottesman, I. I. (1991). *Schizophrenia genesis: The origins of madness*. NY: W. H. Freeman and Company.

Green, M. F. (2001). *Schizophrenia revealed: From neurons to social interactions*. New York: Norton.

Gregg, G. S. (1995). Multiple identities and the integration of personality. *Journal of Personality*, *63*, 617–641.

Greig, T. C., Bryson, G. J. and Bell, M. D. (2004). Theory of mind performance in schizophrenia: Diagnostic, symptoms and neuropsychological correlates. *Journal of Nervous and Mental Disease*, *192*, 12–18.

Gunderson, J. G., Frank A. F., Katz, H. M., Vannicelli, M. L., Frosch, J. P. and Knapp, P. H. (1984). Effects of psychotherapy in schizophrenia: II. Comparative outcome of two forms of treatment. *Schizophrenia Bulletin*, *10*, 564–598.

Habermas, J. (1981). *Theory of communicative action: Vol. 2.* Boston, MA: Beacon Press.

Habermas, J. (1988). *Postmetaphysical thinking.* Cambridge, MA: MIT University Press.

Harding, C. M., Zubin, J. and Strauss, J. (1992). Chronicity in schizophrenia. *British Journal of Psychiatry*, *161*(Suppl. 18), 27–37.

Harrow, M., Grossman, L. S., Herbener, E. S. and Davies, E. W. (2000). Ten-year outcome: Patients with schizoaffective disorders, schizophrenia, affective disorders and mood-incongruent psychotic symptoms. *British Journal of Psychiatry*, *117*, 421–426.

Hartwell, C. E. (1996). The schizophrenogenic mother concept in American psychiatry. *Psychiatry*, 59, 274–297.

Hegel G. F. (1979). *The phenomenology of spirit.* Oxford: Oxford University Press. Originally published in 1807.

Heidegger, M. (1962). *Being and time.* New York: Harper and Row. (Original Work published in 1927).

Heidegger, M. (1993). What is metaphysics? *Basic writings: Revised and expanded edition.* Ed. David Farrell Krell. San Francisco, CA: Harper Collins. (Original Work published in 1929).

Heinrichs, R. W. (2001). *In search of madness: Schizophrenia and neuroscience.* New York: Oxford University Press.

Herbener, E. S., Harrow, M. and Hill, S. K. (2005). Change in the relationship between anhedonia and functional deficits over a 20-year period in individuals with schizophrenia. *Schizophrenia Research*, *75*, 97–105.

Hermans, H. J. M. (1996a). Opposites in a dialogical self: Constructs as characters. *Journal of Constructive Psychology*, *9*, 1–26.

Hermans, H. J. M. (1996b). Voicing the self: From information processing to dialogical interchange. *Psychological Bulletin*, *119*, 31–50.

Hermans, H. J. M., Rijks, T. I. and Kempen, H. J. G. (1993). Imaginal dialogues in the self: Theory and method. *Journal of Personality*, *61*, 207–236.

Hoffman, H. and Kupper, Z. (2002). Facilitators of psychosocial recovery from schizophrenia. *International Review of Psychiatry*, *14*, 293–302.

Holowka, D. W., King, S., Saheb, D., Puckall, M. and Brunet, A. (2003). Childhood abuse and dissociative symptoms in adult schizophrenia. *Schizophrenia Research*, *60*, 87–90.

Hume, D. (1888). *A treatise of human nature*. Oxford: Oxford University Press. Originally published 1734.

Huttunen, M. O. and Niskanen, P. (1978). Prenatal loss of father and psychiatric disorders. *Archives of General Psychiatry, 34*, 429–431.

James, W. (1897/1956) *The will to believe and other essays in popular philosophy*. New York: Dover Publications.

Jenkins, J. H. (2004). Schizophrenia as a paradigm case for understanding fundamental human processes. In J. H. Jenkins and R. J. Barrett (eds), *Schizophrenia culture and subjectivity* (pp. 29–62). New York: Cambridge University Press.

Jeste, D. V., Symonds, L. L. and Harris, M. J. (1997). Nondementia nonpraecox dementia praecox? Late-onset schizophrenia. *American Journal of Geriatric Psychiatry, 5*, 302–317.

Johnson, M. (1993). *The moral imagination*. Chicago, IL: University of Chicago Press.

Karon, B. P. and Van Denbos, G. R. (1981). *Psychotherapy of schizophrenia: The treatment of choice*. New York: Jason Aronson.

Kendell, R. E., McInneny, K., Juszcak, E. and Bain, M. (2000). Obstetric complications and schizophrenia: Two case control studies based on structured obstetric records. *British Journal of Psychiatry, 176*, 516–526.

Kety, S. S. (1987). The significance of genetic factors in the etiology of schizophrenia: Results from the national study of adoptees in Denmark. *Journal of Psychiatric Research, 12*, 423–429.

Kirkpatrick, B. and Buchanan, R. W. (1990). The neural basis of the deficit syndrome in schizophrenia. *Journal of Nervous and Mental Disease, 178*, 545–555.

Knight, R. P. (1946). Psychotherapy of an adolescent catatonic schizophrenic with mutism. *Psychiatry, 9*, 323–339.

Koehler, K., Guth, W. and Grimm, G (1977) First-rank symptoms of schizophrenia in Schneider-oriented German centers. *Archives of General Psychiatry, 34*, 810–813.

Kraeplin, E. (2002). *Dementia praecox and paraphrenia* (M. Barclay, Trans.). Bristol, UK: Thoemmes Press. (Original work published 1919).

Laing, R. D. (1978). *The divided self*. New York: Penguin Books.

Lally, S. J. (1989). Does being in here mean there is something wrong with me? *Schizophrenia Bulletin, 15*, 253–265.

Lamb, H. R. and Weinberger, L. E. (1998). Persons with severe mental illness in jails and prisons: A review. *Psychiatric Services, 49*, 483–492.

Lee, S., Lee, M. T., Chiu, M. Y. and Kleinman, A. (2005). Experience of social stigma by people with schizophrenia in Hong Kong. *British Journal of Psychiatry, 18*, 153–157.

Leudar, I. and Thomas, P. (2000). *Voices of reason, voices of insanity: Studies of verbal hallucinations*. London, England: Routledge.

Lewine, R., Haden, C., Caudel, J. and Shurett, R. (1997). Sex-onset effects on neuropsychological function in schizophrenia. *Schizophrenia Bulletin, 23*, 51–61.

Link, B. G. (1987). Understanding labeling effects in the area of mental disorders: An assessment of the effects of expectations of rejections. *American Sociological Review*, *52*, 96–112.

Link, B. G., Frances, T. C., Struening, E., Shrout, P. E. and Dohrenwend, B. P. (1989). A modified labeling theory approach to mental disorders: An empirical assessment. *American Sociological Review*, *54*, 400–423.

Link, B. G., Phelan, M., Bresnahan, M., Stueve, A. and Pescosolido, B. A. (1999). Public conceptions of mental illness: Labels, causes, dangerousness and social distance. *American Journal of Public Health*, *89*(9), 1328–1333.

Lysaker, J. T. and Lysaker, P. H. (2005). Being interrupted: The self and schizophrenia. *Journal of Speculative Philosophy*, *19*, 1–22.

Lysaker, P. H. and Hammersly, J. (2006). Association of delusions and lack of cognitive flexibility with social anxiety in schizophrenia spectrum disorders. *Schizophrenia Research*, *86*, 137–143.

Lysaker, P. H. and Lysaker, J. T. (2006). Psychotherapy and schizophrenia: An analysis of requirements of an individual psychotherapy for persons with profoundly disorganized selves. *Journal of Constructivist Psychology*, *19*, 171–189.

Lysaker, P. H., Beattie, N. L., Strasburger, A. M. and Davis, L. W. (2005). Reported history of child sexual abuse in schizophrenia: Associations with heightened symptom levels and poorer participation over four months in vocational rehabilitation. *Journal of Nervous and Mental Disease*, *193*, 790–795.

Lysaker, P. H., Bell, M. D., Bioty, S. M. and Zito, W. (1996). Performance on the Wisconsin Card Sorting Test as a predictor of rehospitalization in schizophrenia. *Journal of Nervous and Mental Disease*, *183*, 319–321.

Lysaker, P. H., Bryson, G. J. and Bell, M. D. (2002). Insight and work performance in schizophrenia. *Journal of Nervous and Mental Disease*, *190*(3), 142–146.

Lysaker, P. H., Bryson, G. J., Lancaster, R., Evans, J. D. and Bell, M. D. (2003). Insight in schizophrenia: Associations with executive function and coping style. *Schizophrenia Research*, *59*, 41–47.

Lysaker, P. H., Buck, K. D. and Hammoud, K. (2007). Psychotherapy and schizophrenia: An analysis of requirements of individual psychotherapy with persons who experience manifestly barren or empty selves. *Psychology and Psychotherapy*, *30*, 377–387.

Lysaker, P. H., Buck, K. D. and Ringer, J. (2007). The recovery of metacognitive capacity in schizophrenia across thirty two months of individual psychotherapy: A case study. *Psychotherapy Research*, *17*, 713–720.

Lysaker, P. H., Johannesen, J. K. and Lysaker, J. T. (2005). Schizophrenia and the experience of intersubjectivity as threat. *Phenomenology and the Cognitive Science*, *4*, 335–352.

Lysaker, P. H., Lancaster, R. S., Davis, L. and Clements, C. A. (2003) Patterns of neurocognitive deficits and unawareness of illness in schizophrenia. *Journal of Nervous and Mental Disease*, 191, 38–45.

Lysaker, P. H., Meyer, P. S., Evans, J. D., Clements, C. A. and Marks, K. A. (2001). Childhood sexual trauma and psychosocial functioning in adults with schizophrenia. *Psychiatric Services*, 52(11), 1485–1488.

Lysaker, P. H., Roe, D. and Yanos, P. T. (2007). Toward understanding the insight paradox: Internalized stigma moderates the association between insight and social functioning, hope and self-esteem among people with schizophrenia spectrum disorders. *Schizophrenia Bulletin*, 33, 192–199.

MacIntrye, A. (1984). *After virtue*, 2nd edn. Notre Dame, IN: Notre Dame University Press.

MacKenzie, C. (2000). Imagining oneself otherwise. In: Catriona Mackenzie and Natalie Stoljar (eds), Relational autonomy (pp. 124–150). New York: Oxford University Press.

Mallet, R., Leff, J., Bhugra, D., Pang, D. and Zhao, J. H. (2002). Social environment, ethnicity and schizophrenia. A case control study. *Social Psychiatry and Psychiatric Epidemiology*, 37, 329–335.

Markowitz, F. E. (1998). The effects of stigma on the psychological well-being and life satisfaction of persons with mental illness. *Journal of Health and Social Behavior*, 39, 335–347.

Martin, J. K., Pescosolido, B. A. and Tuch, S. A. (2000). Of fear and loathing: The role of disturbing behavior, labels and causal attributions in shaping public attitudes toward persons with mental illness. *Journal of Health and Social Behavior*, 41(2), 208–233.

McGlashan, T. H. (1998). The profiles of clinical deterioration in schizophrenia. *Journal of Psychiatric Research*, 32, 133–141.

McGlashan, T. H. and Hoffman, R. E. (2000). Schizophrenia as a disorder of developmentally reduced synaptic connectivity. *Archives of General Psychiatry*, 57, 637–648.

McGrath, J., Saha, S., Welham, J., El Saadi, O., MacCauley, C. and Chant, D. (2004). A systematic review of the incidence of schizophrenia: The distribution of rates and the influence of sex, urbanicity, migrant status and methodology. *BMC Psychiatry*, 2, 13.

Mechanic, D., McAlpine, D., Rosenfield, S. and Davis, D. (1994). Effects of illness attribution and depression on the quality of life among persons with serious mental illness. *Social Science and Medicine*, 39, 155–164.

Mednick, S. A., Machon, R. A., Huttunen, M. O. and Bonett, D. (1988). Adult schizophrenia following premature exposure to an influenza epidemic. *Archives of General Psychiatry*, 45, 189–192.

Minkowski, E. (1987). The essential disorder underlying schizophrenia and schizophrenic thought. In J. Cutting (ed.), *The clinical roots of the schizophrenic concept*. Cambridge: Cambridge University Press. (Original work published 1927).

Mishara, A. L. (1995). Narrative and psychotherapy: The phenomenology of healing. *American Journal of Psychotherapy*, 49, 180–195.

Mishara, A. L. (1997). Binswanger. In *Encyclopedia of phenomenology* (pp. 62–66). Dordrecht: Kluwer Academy Press.

Mishara, A. L. (2001). On Wolfgang Blankenburg, common sense and schizophrenia. *Philosophy, Psychiatry and Psychology, 8,* 317–322.

Mishara, A. L. (2004). Disconnection of the external and internal in the conscious experience of schizophrenia: Phenomenological, literary and neuroanatomical archaeologies of self. *Philisophica, 73,* 87–126.

Mishara, A. L. (2005). Body self and its narrative representation in schizophrenia: Does the body scheme concept help establish a core deficit? In H. De Prester and V. Knockaert (eds), *Body image and body schema* (pp. 127–152). Amsterdam: John Benjamins.

Mishler, E. and Waxler, N. (1968). *Family processes and schizophrenia.* New York: New York Science House.

Mortensen, P. B., Pedersen, C. B., Westergaard, T., Wohlfahrt, J., Ewald, H., Mors, O. *et al.* (1999). Effects of family history and place and season of birth on the risk of schizophrenia. *New England Journal of Medicine, 340*(8), 603–608.

Mosher, L. (1999). Sotaria and other alternatives to acute hospitalization. *Journal of Nervous and Mental Disease, 187,* 142–149.

Mueser, K. T., Salyers, M. P., Rosenberg, S. D., Goodman, L. A., Essock, S. M., Osher F. C. *et al.* (2003). Interpersonal trauma and PTSD in severe mental illness. *Schizophrenia Bulletin, 30,* 45–59.

Mueser, K. T., Yarnold, P. R., Levinson, D. F., Singh, H., Bellack, A. S., Kee, K. *et al.* (1990). Prevalence of substance abuse in schizophrenia: Demographic and clinical correlates. *Schizophrenia Bulletin, 16*(1), 31–56.

Nagel, T. (1974). 'What is it like to be a bat?' *Philosophical Review,* 83, 435–50.

Nagel, T. (1986). *The view from nowhere.* New York: Oxford University Press.

Nayani, T. H. and David, A. S. (1996). The auditory hallucination: A phenomenological survey. *Psychological Medicine, 26,* 177–189.

Neimeyer, R. A. (1994). The role of client-generated narratives in psychotherapy. *Journal of Constructivist Psychology, 7,* 229–242.

Neimeyer, R. A. and Raskin, J. D. (2000). *Constructions of Disorder: Meaning-making frameworks for psychotherapy.* Washington, DC: APA Press.

Nelson, M. D., Saykin, A. J., Flashman, and L. A., Riordan, H. J. (1998). Hippocampal volume reduction in schizophrenia as assessed by magnetic resonance imaging. *Archives of General Psychiatry, 55,* 433–454.

Nietzsche, F. (1966). *Beyond good and evil.* New York: Random House. (Original work published 1886).

Nietzsche, F. (1974). *The gay science.* New York: Random House. (Original work published 1887).

Olfson, M., Marcus, S. C., Wilk, J. and West, J. C. (2006). Awareness of illness and nonadherence to antipsychotic medications among persons with schizophrenia. *Psychiatric Services, 57*(2), 205–211.

Oliver, K. (2002). Subjectivity as responsivity: The ethical implications of dependency. In: Kittay, E.F. and Feder, E.K. (eds), *The subject of care: Feminist perspectives on dependency* (pp. 322–333). Lanham, CO: Rowman and Littlefield Publishers, Inc.

Olney, J. W. and Farber, M. D. (1995). Glutamate receptor dysfunction and schizophrenia. *Archives of General Psychiatry, 52,* 998–1007.

Page, S. (1983). Psychiatric stigma: Two studies of behavior when the chips are down. *Canadian Journal of Community Mental Health, 2,* 13–19.

Pallanti, S., Quercioli, L. and Hollander, E. (2004). Social anxiety in outpatients with schizophrenia: A relevant cause of disability. *American Journal of Psychiatry, 161*(1), 53–58.

Pao-Nie, P. (1979). On the formation of schizophrenic symptoms. *International Journal of Psychoanalysis, 58,* 389–401.

Parnas, J. and Handest, P. (2003). Phenomenology of anomalous self-experience in early schizophrenia. *Comprehensive Psychiatry, 44,* 121–134.

Penn, D. L., Spaulding, W., Reed, D., Sullivan, M., Mueser, K. T. and Hope, D. A. (1997). Cognition and social functioning in schizophrenia. *Psychiatry: Interpersonal and Biological Processes, 60*(4), 281–291.

Pescosolido, B. A. (1997). Beyond rational choice: The social dynamics of how people seek help. *American Journal of Sociology, 97,* 1096–1138.

Pescosolido, B. A., Monahan, J., Link, B. G., Stueve, A. and Kikuzawa, S. (1999). The public's view of the competence, dangerousness and need for legal coercion of persons with mental health problems. *American Journal of Public Health, 89*(9), 1339–1345.

Phelan, J. C., Link, B. G., Stueve, A. and Pescosolido, B. A. (2000). Public conceptions of mental illness in 1950 and 1996: What is mental illness and is it to be feared? *Journal of Health and Social Behavior, 41*(2), 188–207.

Porte, J. and Morris, S. (eds) (2001). *Emerson's prose and poetry.* New York: W. W. Norton and Company.

Read, J., Perry, B. D., Moskowitz, A. and Connolly, J. (2001). The contribution of early traumatic events to schizophrenia in some patients: A traumagenic neurodevelopmental model. *Psychiatry, 64,* 319–345.

Rector, N. A. and Beck, A. T. (2002). Cognitive therapy for schizophrenia: From conceptualization to intervention. *Canadian Journal of Psychiatry, 47,* 39–48.

Ritsher, J. B., Otilingam, P. G. and Grajales, M. (2003). Internalized stigma of mental illness: Psychometric properties of a new measure. *Psychiatry Research, 121,* 31–49.

Roe, D. (2001). Exploring the relationship between the person and the disorder among individuals hospitalized for psychosis. *Psychiatry, 62,* 372–380.

Roe, D. and Ben-Yishai, A. (1999). Exploring the relationship between the person and the disorder among individuals hospitalized for psychosis. *Psychiatry, 62,* 370–380.

Roe, D. and Davidson, L. (2005). Self and narrative in schizophrenia: Time to author a new story. *Journal of Medical Humanities*, *31*, 89–94.

Roe, D. and Kravetz, S. (2003). Different ways of being aware of and acknowledging a psychiatric disability: A multifunctional narrative approach to insight into mental disorder. *Journal of Nervous and Mental Disease*, *191*, 417–424.

Rorty, R. (1989). *Contingency, irony* and *solidarity.* Cambridge: Cambridge University Press.

Rosen, J. (1947). The treatment of schizophrenic psychosis by direct analytic therapy. *Psychiatric Quarterly*, *21*, 3–37.

Rosenfield, S. (1997). Labeling mental illness: The effects of received services and perceived stigma on life satisfaction. *American Sociological Review*, *62*, 660–672.

Ross, C. A. Anderson, G. and Clark, P. (1994). Childhood abuse and the positive symptoms of schizophrenia. *Hospital and Community Psychiatry*, *45*(5), 489–491.

Rudge, T. and Morse, K. (2001). Re-awakening?: A discourse analysis of the recovery from schizophrenia after medication change. *Australian and New Zealand Journal of Mental Health Nursing*, *10*, 66–76.

Sartre, J. P. (1956). *Being and nothingness.* New York: Philosophical Library.

Sass, L. A. (1992). Heidegger, schizophrenia and the ontological difference. *Philosophical Psychology*, *5*, 109–133.

Sass, L. A. (2003). *Madness and modernism: Insanity in the light of modern art, literature and thought.* Cambridge, MA: Harvard University Press.

Saykin, A. J., Gur, R. C., Gur, R. E., Mozley, P. D., Mozley, L. H., Resnick, S. M. *et al.* (1991). Neuropsychological function in schizophrenia: Selective impairment in memory and learning. *Archives of General Psychiatry*, *48*, 618–624.

Schwartz, M., Wiggins, O., Naudin, J. and Spitzer, M. (2005). Rebuilding reality: A phenomenology of aspects of chronic schizophrenia. *Phenomenology and the Cognitive Sciences*, *4*, 91–115.

Searles, H. (1965). *Collected papers of schizophrenia and related subjects.* New York: International Universities Press.

Selzer, M. A. and Schwartz, F. (1994). The continuity of personality in schizophrenia. *Journal of Psychotherapy Practice and Research*, *3*, 313–324.

Sensky, T., Turkington, D., Kingdom, D., Scott, J. L., Scott, J., Siddle, R., Carrol, M. and Barnes, T. R. E. (2000). A randomized controlled trial of cognitive behavioral therapy for persistent symptoms in schizophrenia resistant to medication. *Archives of General Psychiatry*, *57*, 165–172.

Solano, J. J. R. and De Chavez, M. G. (2000). Premorbid personality disorders in schizophrenia. *Schizophrenia Research*, *44*(2), 137–144.

Sosowsky, L. (1980). Explaining the increased arrest rate among mental patients: A cautionary note. *American Journal of Psychiatry*, *137*(12), 1602–1604.

Stanghellini, G. (2004). *Disembodied spirits and deanimated bodies.* Oxford: Oxford University Press.

Startup, M. (1997). Awareness of own and others' schizophrenic illness. *Schizophrenia Research*, *26*(2–3), 203–211.

Strauss, J. S., Hafez, H., Lieberman, P. and Harding, C. M. (1985). The course of psychiatric disorders III: Longitudinal principles. *American Journal of Psychiatry*, *142*, 289–296.

Strawson, G. (2004). Against narrativity. *Ratio*, *17*, 428–452.

Strawson, P (1974). *Freedom and resentment*. London: Metheun and Co. Ltd.

Sullivan, H. S. (1962). *Schizophrenia as a human process*. New York: Norton.

Susser, E. S. and Lin, S. P. (1992). Schizophrenia after prenatal exposure to the Dutch hunger winter of 1944–1945. *Archives of General Psychiatry*, *49*(12), 983–988.

Swindle, R., Heller, K., Pescosolido, B. A. and Kikuzawa, S. (2000). Responses to nervous breakdowns in America over a 40-year period: Mental health policy implications. *American Psychologist*, *55*(7), 740–749.

Tarrier, N. and Wykes, T. (2004). Is there evidence that cognitive behaviour therapy is an effective treatment for schizophrenia? A cautious or cautionary tale? *Behaviour Research and Therapy*, *42*, 1377–1401.

Tarrier, N., Kinney, C., McCarthy, E., Humphreys, L., Wittkowski, A. and Morris, J. (2000). Two-year follow-up of cognitive–behavioral therapy and supportive counseling in the treatment of persistent symptoms in chronic schizophrenia. *Journal of Consulting and Clinical Psychology*, *68*, 917–922.

Thompson, E. H. (1988). Variations in the self-concept of young adult chronic patients: Chronicity reconsidered. *Hospital and Community Psychiatry*, *39*, 771–775.

Torgalsboen, A. K. and Rund, B. J. (1998). Full recovery from schizophrenia in the long term: A ten-year follow-up of eight former schizophrenia patients. *Psychiatry*, *61*, 20–34.

Torrey, E. F. (2001). *Surviving schizophrenia*, 4th edn. New York: Harper Collins.

Torrey, E. F., Bowler, A. E., Rawlings, R. and Terrazas, A. (1993). Seasonality of schizophrenia and stillbirths. *Schizophrenia Bulletin*, *19*, 557–562.

van Os, J., Hanssen, M., Bijl, R. V. and Vollebergh, W. (2001). Prevalence of psychotic disorder and community level of psychotic symptoms: An urban–rural comparison. *Archives of General Psychiatry*, *58*(7), 663–668.

Wahl, O. F. (1999). Mental health consumers' experience of stigma. *Schizophrenia Bulletin*, *25*, 467–478.

Wahl, O. F. and Harman, C. R. (1989). Family views of stigma. *Schizophrenia Bulletin*, *15*, 131–134.

Walker, E. F. D. and Diforio, D. (1997). Schizophrenia: A neural diathesis stress model. *Psychological Review*, *104*, 667–685.

Warner, R., Taylor, D., Powers, M. and Hyman, R. (1989). Acceptance of the mental illness label by psychotic patients: Effects on functioning. *American Journal of Orthopsychiatry*, *59*, 389–409.

Weiden, P. and Havens, L. (1994). Psychotherapeutic management techniques in the treatment of outpatients with schizophrenia. *Hospital and Community Psychiatry, 45*, 549–555.

Wexler, M. (1971). Schizophrenia as conflict and deficiency. *Psychoanalytic Quarterly, 40*, 83–100.

Whitaker, R. (2002). *Mad in America*. New York: Perseus.

Williams, C. C. and Collins, A. A. (1999). Defining new frameworks for psychosocial interventions. *Psychiatry, 62*, 61–78.

Wright, E. R., Gronfein, W. P. and Owens, T. J. (2000). Deinstitutionalization, social rejection and the self esteem of former mental patients. *Journal of Health and Social Behavior, 41*, 68–90.

Young, S. L. and Ensign, D. S. (1999). Exploring recovery from the perspective of persons with psychiatric disabilities. *Psychosocial Rehabilitation Journal, 22*, 219–231.

Zakzanis, K. K. and Heinrichs, R. W. (1999). The frontal executive hypothesis in schizophrenia: A quantitative review. *Journal of the International Neuropsychological Society, 5*, 556–566.

Zubin, J. and Spring, B. (1977). Vulnerability: A new view of schizophrenia. *Journal of Abnormal Psychology, 86*(2), 103–126.

Index